Love is
The Answer

I0157309

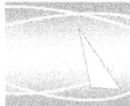

Blue Ocean Publishing

Love is The Answer

Published by Blue Ocean Publishing
St John's Innovation Centre
Cambridge CB4 0WS
United Kingdom

http://www.blueoceanpublishing.biz

A catalogue record for this book is available from the British Library.

ISBN 978-1-907527-32-6

First published in the United Kingdom in 2017 by Blue Ocean Publishing.

For my family, friends, colleagues, clients and lovers.
Thank you for teaching me so much about Love.

And for Mark.
I meet a lot of people, and many of them touch my heart,
but very few of them touch my soul as you have.

A percentage of the profits from this book are being donated to the Ice Warrior Project; an on-going, environmentally-focused project dedicated to engaging ordinary people from all walks of life to become modern-day polar explorers and carry out crucial data gathering under the guidance of the world's leading scientists.

The latest flagship expedition is to the last unexplored region of the North Pole, 'the Northern Pole of Inaccessibility'. Rare Arctic wolves and polar bears are being counted and studied by the expedition teams, and the real depth of the melting Arctic sea ice is being measured on behalf of NASA, the UK's Royal Aeronautical Society and the UK's Meteorological Office. If you care at all about our environment and our planet, please support this citizen-science endeavour at *www.ice-warrior.com*

Acknowledgements

No-one writes a book alone. It may feel that way sometimes in those random hours of writing when seemingly only Facebook and online forums are awake, but the reality is that many people, ideas and voices create the words that you, the reader, finally read on the page. Neither are these ideas and imprints linear; sometimes years and continents divide them until they are all finally sewn together into something meaningful. So my first thanks are to those people, ideas and voices who will never know the value, influence and impact they had on me.

Special thanks are due to the amazing Sarah Frossell who understands more about good writing and the structure of language than anyone else I have ever met. Thank you for being such a wonderful friend over the years. I value your approach, your contributions and your support more than words can express.

Particular thanks are also due to my friend and colleague, Paul. It was thoughts about his leadership style which led me to develop the Corporate Love Model in Chapter 8. Of all the people I know, Paul is probably the most pragmatically critical and least likely person to ever purchase or read a book about Love, especially Love in the workplace. So I have been able to use him as a mental benchmark to keep my thinking on the right path. If my prose became too flowery or I lost my way in my approach, it was Paul who generously and supportively nudged me back on track.

Whilst I was writing this book for you I presented the Corporate Love Model in public for the first time. It was at the British Psychological Society's Division of Occupational Psychology Conference in the January of 2017 in Liverpool, UK. The model was so well received, and the feedback so positive and so enthusiastic, that it really gave me the strength and the courage to carry on and keep going.

Writing can often be a very insular, even lonely, job, and there have been times when I've wondered whether I'm really on the right path.

It seems that I am, and also that there is a real and genuine need for someone to raise their head above the parapet and champion Corporate Love, Love in the workplace, Authentic Loving Leadership, Compassionate Leadership and Leading with Love. They are all the same thing; they simply use a language people are more familiar, and comfortable, with. I'm up for the challenge, and I hope that in your own way, you will join me on the journey. It's a strange thing, but it's beginning to feel like a Dragon's Quest. Except that we're not slaying anything. Rather, we're bringing Love, light and understanding to a dark corporate landscape, where profit and greed have ruled for too long.

As a last word, many other friends and colleagues have also contributed to the book, often in ways they were unaware of at the time. A useful question or conversation, an enquiry as to progress or a suggestion or two. All were hugely beneficial.

My grateful thanks to you all.

Contents

A Special Introduction from the Author

"What is the purpose of life?" the young monk asked his teacher.
"The purpose of life is to live", he replied.

It seems to me that people live their lives in one of two ways. They either embrace life fully, living and learning as much as they can, with enormous courage and with no holds barred, trying everything they can, which often involves experimenting with things like alcohol, drugs, love, addictions, dangerous sports, trauma or near-death experiences. They run headlong into life with their arms and their hearts wide open, living in the moment for the moment, and squeezing every last drop of meaning into their experience of what it is to be human and to be alive. Sometimes in error they die young, which is a terrible tragedy, but at least we can say that they have truly lived.

Or, people hide from life, too scared to embrace it. They watch life pass them by from the sidelines, arms folded keeping everyone at a safe distance. They wish that they had the courage, the bravery and the attitude to grab life with both hands and live fully and whole heartedly, but they are so scared of being hurt, of somehow getting it wrong, or of being ridiculed by others, that they live their lives with their eyes averted and their hearts closed. They worry too much about what other people might think of them and they believe, mistakenly, that they are protecting themselves.

But all their fearful self-protection does is prevent their self-expression and any kind of passionate, fulfilling engagement, and so they live inauthentic lives, imagining what might have been if only they had found the courage to speak out or follow their dreams. Over time they settle for mediocrity, or worse, they withdraw from life, often becoming increasingly cynical, negative or depressed. They die with regrets, never having fully lived, never having found their passion or achieved their full potential.

I've written this book for both kinds of people. If you are the first kind of person this book will give you new knowledge, new information and a new energy regarding the meaning of life and what it is to experience a full and happy existence on this beautiful planet of ours. You will find profound insights within its pages, which will make your life more meaningful.

For the second kind of person, if that is you, you will find the permission to live your life differently. You will discover a greater understanding in those pieces of the giant jigsaw puzzle of life that have eluded you so far. You will find greater self-acceptance, more Love, more passion, the potential for joy, and, ultimately, for peace.

"What is my Purpose in Life?" I asked the Universe.
"To help people recreate their futures, in a safe and supportive environment", came the reply.

Do all things with Love.

Fiona Beddoes-Jones, 2017

Prologue

"The best love is the kind that awakens the soul
and makes us reach for more,
that plants a fire in our hearts
and brings peace to our minds"
The Notebook, by Nicholas Sparks, Novelist.

Readers often seem to wonder where writers get their ideas from. I myself am always fascinated to go to writers' workshops and hear other writers describe their ideas and their writing process and the people who have inspired them. It's often said that you can't become a great writer without first becoming a great reader, and from that perspective I owe a huge debt to the authors of all of the self-help, self-development and spiritual awareness books which I have read and re-read over the past 35 years or so.

Our spirituality and our self- awareness seem to me to be something into which we grow, and, if we are really lucky, rather like baking a cake with ingredients from the cupboard which we happened to have all along, our growth will coincide with our desire and ability to support, nurture and cherish others so that we can share our experiences and what we've learned in ways which are also useful to them.

I have always been fascinated by people, by what makes us similar to or different from others and by how our thinking influences our language and behaviours, the lives we lead and the relationships that we have. It was this fascination that led to me becoming a psychologist, mediator and professional coach, and it was my experiences with meeting and speaking with thousands of people and listening to those issues and problems that were adversely affecting their personal and professional lives which made me realise two very fundamental things.

The first thing I realised is that there are two types of people in the world: there are those people who can help and then there are those people who need help. Each and every one of us is both a person who can help and a person who needs help, and, somewhat confusingly, often at the same time. You will find more about this in Chapter 3 where we explore Healthy Self-Love, and also in Chapter 9, where we will be exploring the ways in which Love is The Answer in more depth, and from a variety of different perspectives.

The second fundamental truth I realised, and it took me a long time to understand it, is that in every situation that someone described or discussed with me, whether that was within the context of personal life coaching, executive coaching at work, mediation, counselling or simply supporting a friend through a tough time, where people were involved, even if it was just one person, that what needed untangling and understanding was something about relationships. And where relationships are involved, then Love really is The Answer.

This fundamental truth, about Love being The Answer, holds true especially if the only person in the relationship is you. Arguably, the most important relationship that we ever have is not with our parents or primary care givers, but with ourselves.

This is true when things are going well for us. However it becomes even more apparent, and even more important, when things aren't going so well for us. The stories and case studies in Chapter 9 will really bring these fundamental truths to life for you, and they will enable you to reflect on what you might do if you were to find yourself in the same situation. I can guarantee that your personal thoughts and responses will be insightful and that your own self-awareness and self-understanding will increase as a result.

Interestingly, sometimes the people I worked with in my coaching, counselling and mediation roles needed to love themselves a little bit more. Sometimes the opposite was true; they needed to love other people more. Frequently however it was both, because if we need to give genuine understanding, compassion and forgiveness to others, very often, we also need to give it to ourselves.

Occasionally, I would meet someone who needed to love themselves less. In my experience as a Chartered Psychologist I know that, while true psychological narcissism is quite rare, simple selfishness or a lack of consideration for others are not. This really is an unhappy combination, because it means that people are not being their 'best selves'. They are denying themselves the gifts of kindness, compassion and of loving others and they are also denying themselves the gift of genuine and appropriate self-love.

However, the good news is that a greater understanding of ourselves and others, and more acceptance and forgiveness of both ourselves and others, are the cornerstones of the healing process, and this process can begin at any age.

So it was these realisations, crafted over years of life and experience, combined with an understanding of how loving and being loved fundamentally affects us at a cellular level, both biologically and neurologically, which eventually meant that I simply had to put pen to paper and start writing.

Even though Love is all around us, there still needs to be more Love in our world, and there definitely needs to be more Love, kindness, emotional generosity, compassion and understanding in the workplace, which is why I have included Chapter 8 on Corporate Love: Loving and Leadership. Here you will find The Corporate Love Model and the results of some original research conducted in the UK in the autumn of 2016 on Love in the workplace. For reasons that will become obvious as you read on, I labelled it as leadership style research. I didn't want people becoming confused and thinking that I was researching sex in the stationary cupboard!

Primarily written for personal development, this probably isn't the kind of book which many leaders or managers might pick up and read;

but perhaps they need to. After all, it's the leaders and managers who set the tone in their organizations. Whether they like it or not, socially and culturally, leaders and managers are the role models other people will copy, especially younger people. So, like good or bad parenting, whatever our leaders and managers do, they are effectively giving other people permission to do it too.

Do you have a leader or manager at work who you think needs to understand themselves a bit better? Or whom you feel needs to lead and manage you more effectively by being more considerate, compassionate or understanding? If you do, I would suggest having a small collection to get them a copy of this book. You never know, you may find that it helps.

So, to give you an overview of the things we are going to explore together, in Chapter 1 we begin by considering the question, "What is Love?" There is no simple and easy answer as Love is multi-faceted and in everyday linguistic parlance people now use the word 'love' to describe many things and many different depths of feelings for someone or something. Chapter 1 also explores our historical and modern passion for Love.

Chapter 2 explains the neurology, biology and psychology of Love. We really are 'wired for love' from a physical, biological and chemical perspective, and also from a neurological perspective. Understanding these things and pulling together all of the strands from what we currently know about the 'mind/body link' of the vagus nerve, oxytocin and our neurology, will help you to understand why we crave Love, how Love and loving can heal us at a cellular level and how losing Love, or a lack of Love is fundamentally dangerous to our health and for our well-being. In other words, Chapter 2 explains our body's need for Love.

The ancient Greeks had words for seven different kinds of Love. But over 3,000 years, our world and society have changed, and our understanding of Love and relationships has also altered.

Sociologists and Social Psychologists call such changes, 'Cultural Relativism'. So in Chapter 3 we explore the 10 different kinds of Love that we now experience in our modern-day world.

Chapter 4 contains the Love Audit. This is your opportunity to identify and map out how much of each of the 10 different types of modern Love you currently have in your life. You will also have the opportunity to think about whether this is the ideal balance for you or whether you are, in fact, out-of-balance regarding your unique levels of the kinds of Love that you intuitively know would be your ideal combination. This chapter is very powerful and will provide you with fundamental insights into your own 'Love Map'; what you have and what you need.

It's all very well completing your Love Audit in Chapter 4 and understanding whether your desires and need for Love are currently being met. But what can you do if you discover that you are out-of-balance and that, in order to be happier, you will need to change some things? Chapter 5 takes a look at how you can bring more of each of the 10 different kinds of Love into your life and helps you to think through the next steps that you might want to take so that you can feel more emotionally in-balance and more fulfilled; thereby improving your physical and mental health.

Sometimes through no fault of our own, we lose Love. Sometimes we lose Love because elements of our thinking or behaviour become incompatible with others. Sometimes we lose Love because elements of other people's thinking or behaviour have become incompatible with what we need in our lives at that specific time. And sometimes we lose Love because what was once good Love goes bad. If any of these things have ever happened to you, you will know how devastating it is to lose Love, whatever the cause. Chapter 6 explains the chemical, biological and neurological reasons why losing Love or bad Love is so distressing and ultimately destructive to our physical and mental well-being, and what we can do to minimise its damaging effects. We also explore the concept of 'Tough Love' and explain how we can use Tough Love *with Love*, so that we are acting from a place of love, kindness and compassion, and not from a place of anger, fear, pain or revenge.

Chapter 7, How Love Can Heal You and Heal Your Life, may be one of the most important chapters you read. It was almost Chapter 2, but I wanted to be able to build on what we've learned about the 10 different kinds of Love, and I also wanted us to be able to build on our new understanding of the psychobiology and neurology of Love. Knowing that something is important is a good thing, but understanding why it's important and how it affects us is fundamental to how we prioritise and manage our daily lives.

Love does affect us, there's no doubt about that. It affects all of us, all of the time. It affects our moods and our emotions. It affects our thinking and behaviour. It fundamentally affects us at a cellular level, which is why good loving is so regenerative, and bad loving is so harmful. There is even new evidence to suggest that loving well can ward off the effects of Alzheimer's and dementia and help us to live longer.

There's a slight change of pace in the next chapter. Moving away from love and loving at a personal level, the focus in Chapter 8 is on the workplace and is called The Corporate Love Model: Loving and Leadership. Corporate culture is based on the beliefs and values of the senior executive team and influences all elements of an employee's working experience, from the internal language that is used, to the unwritten psychological contracts that exist between people in the workplace.

Some corporate cultures are more loving and giving, generous, compassionate and supportive than others. Why is that, and how does corporate culture influence productivity, profitability and people's well-being? The Corporate Love Model identifies four different kinds of corporate culture based on the two axis of Conditional and Unconditional Love with Masculine and Feminine Leadership Style. Which is your preferred style and does it match the Corporate Love culture you are currently working in? This chapter also includes the results of some research on loving and leadership that I conducted in the UK in the autumn of 2016.

The Case Studies and vignettes in Chapter 9 really bring the book to life. All the stories are of real people and I would ask you to consider the question, *"In what ways is Love The Answer here?"* As is so often the case, there will be more than one possible response to the issues that are presented, and the ways you react will give you further insights into both your personal Love Map and also into your own Corporate Love Leadership Style preference.

The book closes with an Epilogue where I summarise the thinking in the book and share with you some next steps and my hopes for your future. Here you will also find some suggestions as to what you might want to consider doing next if any parts of the book have particularly resonated with you, and if you have decided that you would like to make some changes to recreate your future in a safe and supportive environment.

Chapter 1

What is Love?

"You live that you may learn to love,
you love that you may learn to live.
No other lesson is required of you"
The Book of Mirdad, by Mikha'il Na'ima, Lebanese Philosopher.

Love, it seems, is all around us. It's in the language of our songs and in the words of our stories. It's completely embedded within our culture, to such an extent that the universal symbol for Love, a heart, is sometimes drawn into the froth on our coffee. In our shops, anything heart-shaped is likely to sell faster and more often than any other shape. Many of us collect heart-shaped objects and images, often with quotes about love embedded within them, and thoughts about loving and being loved often appear unbidden in our heads. So what's going on and why has our human obsession with loving and being loved endured for millennia?

There are many thousands of books written about Love, especially within the shelves of the self-help, personal psychology and personal development sections. Interestingly though, their focus is often a singular one; ideas on Romantic Love for example: how to find Romantic Love and keep it, how to be 'The One', what to look for in a romantic life partner, etc. Or, they focus on another specific kind of Love; Self-Love for example, written for the many people who somehow don't quite know how to love themselves enough and have lost their way. Family Love, managing teenagers and other familial challenges are another popular area many of us need help with, as every generation has to learn about themselves and how to manage their emotions and their relationships in an increasingly complex and difficult world.

This book is slightly different to any book about Love that you may have come across before. It explores the question, *"What is Love?"*

from the multiple perspectives of philosophy, psychology, biology and neuroscience, and interweaves them together in a way which will change your understanding of what it means to Love and be Loved.

Love really is good for us, in all kinds of ways. We don't need to be 'in Love' romantically with someone to feel the benefits of Love and loving, although for most of us, that is probably one of the most familiar ways through which we will experience it. One of the other most common ways we find Love is in the profound Love that we have for our children, especially when they are young and need us so very much. Our experience of such loving, both Romantic and Familial are universal. In our modern world we experience the same feelings and emotions today as our ancestors did millennia ago, and the Romantic and Familial Love we feel in the West is arguably the same as the Love felt by every other race, tribe or community world-wide regardless of language, creed or colour.

To Love and to need Love is profoundly human. Love and loving are also profoundly healing. This is equally true whether we are the person doing the loving, or whether we are the person being loved. Perhaps it is because the very acts of 'Falling in Love' and being 'In Love' with someone Romantically, are one of the easiest ways to experience the emotional and physical benefits of Love and loving, that so many of us crave the experience.

Wouldn't it be wonderful if we could fall in Love with life and living and the world around us? If only we could fall in Love with our own lives we wouldn't be so reliant on someone or something else, outside of ourselves, to make us feel loving or loved.

It's my deepest hope that this book will teach you how to do just that, or at least open up a world of possibilities regarding Love and loving that you may not have considered before.

Within the pages of this book you will learn to:

- Recognise what Love is, - it may not be quite what you think.

- Understand how and why Love and loving and being loved nurture us physically as well as emotionally.

- Think about Love differently than you have before.

- Understand passion from a neurobiological perspective.

- Consider Corporate Love and Leadership as they relate to your well-being, engagement and motivation at work.

- Look for Love differently than perhaps you have before.

- Find Love in places that you haven't considered before.

- Understand why the loss of Love affects us so profoundly, and how it can make us physically unwell.

- Recover from losing Love more quickly and more fully than you may have been able to do in the past.

- Understand how Love may be able to ward off dementia, Alzheimer's disease and may help you to live longer.

- Be more loving towards yourself, towards others and within your life, to achieve the personal benefits that Love brings.

- Heal your own life, and that of others, through Love.

So what then is 'Love'?

How do we experience Love? What does it feel like to us inside our bodies when we say that we Love someone or something? And how might being 'in Love' with someone Romantically be different to the feelings of Love we have for our parents, our children or our best friend? We can feel Love, or rather I should say, our heads, our hearts and our bodies will feel the influence of loving via all 10 of the different types of Love described in Chapter 3.

When we do Love, these will be the characteristics that we are most likely to experience.

The Characteristics of 'Love' and of 'Loving'

- Heartfelt and strong emotions.

- Trust and acceptance.

- Passion and excitement.

- Engagement of the vagus nerve, (which may be butterflies in our tummy or a feeling in our solar plexus of complete calm or joy. We will be exploring this more in Chapter 2).

- A desire to *be* loving which also makes us kind and generous.

- Unconditional Regard.

- Respectfulness towards that which we Love.

- Forgiveness, (often in its entirety, however, if we are having to use Tough Love because we have previously been hurt and we are lacking trust, it may just be partial forgiveness with caveats).

- Authenticity.

- Relaxation and a feeling of 'wholeness' or 'completeness'.

- Genuine concern for the well-being and optimal health of those people or things that we Love.

- A willingness to make sacrifices or endure personal hardship if those things will benefit the things or people we Love.

- Very often, but not always, playfulness, depending on our personality type and the degree to which we personally like to have fun and play around.

- Very often, but not always, feelings of protectiveness towards the person, thing or organisation we Love.

- Sometimes, most often in the early stages of loving, an irrational fear of losing that which we Love.

13

Chapter 1: What is Love?

The Characteristics of 'Feeling Loved'

- We feel accepted, completely and fully, for who we are. This allows us, and enables us, to be our authentic selves.

- Engagement of the vagus nerve, generating feelings of excitement, joyfulness, happiness, calm, inner peace, a 'warm fuzzy feeling', or again, maybe 'butterflies' in your tummy.

- The courage to try new things without fear of rejection or failure.

- Feelings of safety, that everything is ok, and will be ok.

- We feel nurtured and protected and supported.

- We want to be 'our best selves' for the person who Loves us.

- We feel respected, 'believed in' and trusted to do our best and be our best, and if we don't quite manage it, then that's ok too.

The Characteristics of Loss, of Losing Love, of Rejection, or when Love is Withheld or Withdrawn (Not everyone will feel all of these. However, they are all common symptoms of the distress and devastation of loss).

- Complete and utter panic.

- Fear, (ranging from mild discomfort to all-consuming terror)

- Feelings of abandonment, rejection, and sometimes guilt, (depending on the circumstances of the loss).

- Obsessive thoughts, (often about what or who we've lost, what we could have done differently, and what we can do to get the Love back), which are often circular, and repetitive in our heads.

- Extreme unhappiness, even wretched misery.

- Depression, (which is both emotional and physical. Our immune systems also become depressed as we will discuss in Chapter 2).

- A significant rise in cortisol, the stress hormone, which is often accompanied by an increase in adrenaline.

- Obsessive compulsive behaviour, (doing things or repeating processes which we think will help us to feel more in control of our thoughts, feelings, and emotions, which we repeat, over and over again in an attempt to self-soothe and feel better).

- Reliance on coping strategies which are often misplaced, (such as alcohol, food, drugs, shopping, dangerous hobbies or other inappropriate but understandable behaviours but ones which may spiral out of control and result in emotional or physical damage).

- A desire to feel nothing emotionally, (as we are in so much emotional pain that feeling nothing is preferable to that).

- Physical responses such as a loss of appetite, disrupted sleep patterns and tears.

- Sometimes we may feel physical pain. Where and how that may manifest itself will depend on each person.

- An inability to get up in the mornings, either because of physical or emotional reasons.

- Somehow becoming constantly 'busy', so we never have a moment to sit and reflect at how unhappy we really are.

- Our immune system also becomes depressed and we may subsequently suffer from general lethargy and a lack of energy, headaches, colds, flu-like symptoms or other real illnesses.

- We may become easily emotionally upset and thrown off-balance by comments or events which we could previously usually have coped with quite easily.

- General feelings of not-coping very well, or at the extreme, thoughts of suicide or self-harming.

- A desire to stay in bed all day, (where it's warm and safe), to 'hibernate' and only emerge when life is somehow magically 'better'; we are fully healed and our world is different and the way we want it to be. (i.e. we have our Love back again).

- Anger. From mild irritation to profound and deep-seated hate. This may be aimed at the world in general or the person or organisation which has 'hurt' us and withdrawn their Love, their protection and support.

- Distrust towards the person or organisation that has hurt us, which may then become generalised in the future to a distrust of all people or all organizations, whom we then expect to behave in the same way as the original perpetrator did.

Reading this list regarding the loss of Love, is it any wonder then that babies and small children, when separated from their primary carers, will exhibit some of the characteristics I've listed? Or that teenagers, when they split up from their 'first true Love', are so distraught? Or spouses, upon discovering that their partner is having an affair and may leave them, feel so utterly devastated?

Divorcees and the bereaved, adults when they are made redundant, friends who fall out and even the owners of a cherished car which is stolen or damaged in some way. The characteristics of loss are the same whether we have lost something or someone we 'love' and feel passionately about as adults or whether we are 18 months old and are inconsolable because we've just lost a much beloved toy.

Critically, and we will explore this much more in Chapter 2, there are real physical changes which take place in the body as a direct result of loss. These biological changes are chemical, affecting our immune system and every cell in the body, including neurological changes which affect our brains. Our thinking profoundly influences our brain chemistry, and our brain chemistry profoundly influences our thinking and subsequent behaviours in a mutual biofeedback mechanism.

Chapter 1: What is Love?

According to the Holmes and Rahe Stress Scale, the 10 most stressful
life events for adults are, in descending order:

1. The death of a spouse   (loss)
2. Divorce   (loss)
3. Marital separation   (loss)
4. Imprisonment   (loss of freedom)
5. Death of a close family member   (loss)
6. Personal injury or illness   (loss of health)
7. Marriage
8. Dismissal from work   (loss of income)
9. Marital reconciliation
10. Retirement   (loss of work)

(For more information, see *www.paindoctor.com*)

Medical doctors recognise the link between stress, distress or some
kind of loss or significant change in circumstances, and any subsequent
physical illness. At first glance, marriage and marital reconciliation
don't appear to be about loss. However, they are a time of great
change and uncertainty, and may, in some people, be accompanied
by feelings of a loss of stability, independence, freedom, or, where a
woman gives up her maiden name to take on the name of her
husband's family, the loss of a much cherished family name and
associated sense of identity. You will find more about recovering
from loss in Chapter 7, How Love Can Heal Your Life.

What is Love? A Note about 'Passion'

Passion is interesting for many reasons, not least of which is that passion seems to echo many of the things that we experience when we feel Love. What I mean by this is that firstly, Love concerns strong feelings and emotions, as does passion. Secondly, we can be passionate about people, things, places, hobbies, pets and our beliefs and principles, just as we can Love those things deeply and profoundly. You might wish to argue here that we don't say that we Love our beliefs or principles, and linguistically that's true. However, what's also true is that some people feel such passion, and such strength of emotion for their religious beliefs and principles, that they are prepared to sacrifice their own lives for them, and in some cases kill and take the lives of others for them.

In a way, that's the fundamental flaw of passion compared to love. Where Love is selfless and giving, passion can be selfish and demanding. The origin of the word passion is early Latin, *'pati'* which means *'suffer'*. The Oxford English dictionary defines passion as, *'A strong and barely controllable emotion, an outburst of emotion, intense sexual love, an intense desire or enthusiasm for something'*, and 'The Passion' as, *'The suffering and death of Jesus on the cross'* in Christian religious doctrine.

The ancient Greeks didn't think very highly of passion either. They considered the passionate love and lust of Eros, what I refer to as Stage 1 Romantic Love, to be immature and unwise. They thought that to be consumed by passion was indeed to suffer and they counselled against it, suggesting that the other forms of Love were somehow of a 'higher' order, presumably because the other forms of love were selfless, giving and supportive rather than selfish, demanding and painful to experience, which passion can sometimes be. Passionate Love can, in some ways, be considered to be akin to madness, or drug addiction, as it occupies the same neural pathways in the brain as narcotics do. But more of that in Chapter 2, The Neurology, Biology and Psychobiology of Love.

Regarding Love, many of us are familiar with feelings of Romantic passion. It will be familiar to many of us regarding the very strong feelings we have towards a romantic and often sexual partner. Or towards someone with whom we want to have a romantic or sexual relationship. So let's look at the characteristics of passion, as some of them are more positive and nurturing than others.

The Characteristics of Passion

- Very strong feelings and emotions.

- Obsessive thoughts; we can't stop thinking about the object of our passion, and the thoughts we have are often circular, they seem to swirl around and around in our heads.

- Thoughts of Love; of being near to, and of 'protecting' the object of our desires.

- Not wanting to share that which we are passionate about; we want to keep it, or them, all to ourselves.

- Thoughts of loss; our 'worst fear' is the loss of that about which we feel so passionately.

- Thoughts of jealousy and possession.

- An inability to think about anything else apart from the thing or person we feel passionately about.

- Being willing to financially pay for, or invest other resources such as our time, in associated activities or material things which relate to that about which we are passionate.

- Not being able to think rationally or clearly

So then, sexual or romantic feelings of passion, when our feelings for someone or something are so strong that thoughts of them consume our waking thoughts and sometimes our dreams too, may be familiar to you. So how does passion manifest itself in relation to the other Types of Love and how is passion beneficial or detrimental to us from the perspective of our emotional, physical and psychological well-being? These are all questions which we will be exploring and answering in future chapters.

Chapter 2

The Neurology and Psychobiology of Love

"Read not to contradict and refute; nor to believe and take for granted; nor to find talk and discourse; but to weigh and consider. Some books are to be tasted, others to be swallowed, and some few to be chewed and digested: that is, some books are to be only read in parts, others to be read, but not curiously, and some few to be read wholly, and with diligence and attention."
Francis Bacon in The Essays.

This chapter will help you to understand why Love has such a powerful hold over us; why we almost seem to be, 'wired for Love'. We will be exploring the science behind our desire to Love and be loved, and the science behind the reasons why we feel such pain when we lose Love. Out of necessity, because it's so complex, I've had to simplify the science in certain places to make it more readable, or to highlight those areas which are most relevant to the effects which Love exerts upon us.

Love is a combination of thoughts, feelings and physical responses that we experience, and it's a strong and powerful emotion. When we experience the emotion of Love we don't just like something, or someone, we LOVE them. These feelings have a profound effect on our neurology, (our brains), and our physiology, (our hearts, and in fact every cell of our bodies). In other words, Love effects our psychobiology at a very profound and fundamental level.

All of the 10 Types of Love effect our psychobiology. This was the main reason I included each of the 10 Types, precisely because when we experience each and every one of them, they change the ways in which we are thinking and feeling; our bodies physically respond to that Love. We also respond neurologically, chemically and on a microcellular level.

21

You might be familiar with the sensation of having 'butterflies in your tummy'. Your physical 'gut feelings' are technically called 'interoceptive sensations' because interoception is the self-awareness of our bodies' physiological responses. Ordinarily, we don't notice them unless there's a significant change in them, or we become uncomfortable in some way. Heart rate is a good example, as are the physical sensations of pain, hunger, thirst, our digestive processes and the regulation of our body temperature.

These interoceptive sensations are sent from our peripheral body to our brain via our afferent nerve receptors, and in a feedback loop system, efferent signals are sent back from our brain to the efferent nerve receptors in our peripheral body. You probably won't be surprised to learn that there are individual differences in how sensitive and self-aware people are to the changes that occur in their bodies. Some people are very self-aware, and other people much less so. We can all learn to become more self-aware of our bodies. Meditation is a common way for people to achieve that.

The Science of Love
Before we explore some of the scientific research which supports our thinking about Love, I want to introduce you to the Vagus Nerve. *Vagus* is Latin for *'wandering'* and our vagus nerve is sometimes known as *The Wandering Nerve* because it is by far the longest of our 12 cranial nerves. It extends from the brainstem at the top of the back of our neck down through our body to almost cradle the stomach. On its journey through the body it extends tendrils into all the major organs and many of the minor ones too.

The idea of human intuition being a physical sense of *gut feeling* was dismissed by science until fairly recently when it was discovered that it's actually the vagus nerve that performs the function of the *mind/body link*. Fear, anxiety, hunger, breathing and relaxation are all fundamentally affected by the vagus nerve. The vagus nerve also regulates the digestion of food in our stomach, which is why when we are upset or scared we often can't eat, and when we are joyously happy or excited we often lose our appetite and can't eat either!

The vagus nerve also has a profound influence on our body's inflammatory and auto-immune responses. The parasympathetic nervous system is responsible for regulating our *rest and digest* response, whereas our sympathetic nervous system is responsible for our *fight/flight/fright* response, where the body is flooded with cortisol, adrenaline and noradrenalin at times of, (perceived), great danger.

The vagus nerve is the major organ of our parasympathetic nervous system and it's involved in sending signals to the brain and the body to release organic chemicals into our bloodstream. The speed and efficiency of our vagus nerve can be measured by how it regulates our heart rate, known as *vagal* tone. More on vagal tone later, as it has profound implications for Love and healing within us.

The psychologist Barbara Fredrickson, originally conceived the idea of Love 2.0 based on the physiological and neurological effects of, what she termed, *'Moments of positive resonance'*, between people. She also investigated the effects on people of practising Buddhist Loving Kindness Meditation. She found that over the course of a seven week period, by practising daily Loving Kindness Meditation, people reported increases in all kinds of positive emotions, particularly love, joy, gratitude, contentment, humour, pride, hope and a greater sense of connection and purpose. All of these things ultimately led to increased feelings of life satisfaction[1].

Loving Kindness Meditation has been shown to assist in the reduction of pain. This makes perfect sense when we think about the science of Love and increases in vagal tone[2]. Loving Kindness Meditation has also been shown to have a beneficial effect on relationships[3]. I've spoken about Loving Kindness Meditation quite a lot. If you are interested in learning more about it, I have included a short guide in Chapter 5, Bringing More Love into Your Life.

How we are 'hard-wired' for Love
Neurologists are constantly making new scientific discoveries about what happens in the brain. They don't always know why things happen or how they happen, just that they do. Maybe one day science will catch up with human evolution! Here are some of the things that we know so far.

Our brains lay down new neural pathways every day of our lives. New learning stimulates this in particular, so the very act of reading this book will be causing tiny electrical impulses within your own brain as new connections are made between your synapses and new neural pathways are created. This is known as 'brain plasticity' and can be thought of as a kind of 'soft-wiring'. If these new neural pathways aren't reused and reinforced, they seem to shrivel and die, in a kind of 'use it or lose it' way.

Of course, this isn't a problem for us as we can lay down new neural pathways and new memories whenever we like, but it does seem to go some way towards explaining why we sometimes struggle with remembering things if we haven't thought about them for a while! However, when we think in a certain way often enough, or about something or someone often enough, these new neural pathways become reinforced again and again, becoming more embedded and easier to access until eventually, they cause structural changes in the brain.

An obvious illustration of this would be learning a new language for example, learning to draw or learning to drive a car. Eventually, the new neural pathways change from being little, rural, one-person-wide footpaths through the forest, into the equivalent of a neural superhighway. That's when our new learning or our new type of thinking has become 'hard-wired' and it results in physical changes in the brain which researchers can actually see on MRI scans.

The practice of daily Loving Kindness Meditation is a perfect example of this where within as short a timescale of just 6 weeks, people who learned to meditate showed significant changes to growth and activity in their left frontal lobes[4]. Meeting a new person and 'Falling in Love' with them, passion in other words, creates the same super-highways in our brains, and that is true whether it's a new romantic partner we can't stop thinking about, or a new baby within our close family. Of course there are other chemical and physiological changes that happen in the body when we fall in Love, which we will explore later on in the chapter.

Mirror neurons are interesting too. They are a special kind of brain cell that exist within our pre-frontal cortex, (amongst other areas). Our pre- frontal cortex is the home of our 'executive thinking', by which I mean our higher-level thinking processes. Problem solving, our 'intelligence', and the assessment of risk and danger all happen here. It's the part of the brain which is thought to be the last to develop, and which doesn't appear to be fully developed until we reach our early twenties, which I always think explains some of the reckless behaviours of teenagers and young adults. We can blame it on their immature brains!

It's our pre-frontal cortex, (along with some other areas), which is 'hijacked' when we experience the rush of cortisol and adrenaline when our fight/flight/fright response is triggered at times of severe and immediate danger. The result of this is that we simply can't think straight. We either don't know which way to turn, like a rabbit stuck in the headlights of a car in the road, or we panic and want to flee the situation, literally running away if we can, or we become aggressive and try to 'fight' our way out of the situation, verbally or physically. As we will go on to explore, for different physiological reasons to do with the effect of self-generated chemical opiates in the brain, passion appears to have the same effect on us. We simply lose all logical reason and can't think straight then either.

The special brain cells are called 'mirror neurons' because they are activated in normal functioning adults and children to 'mirror' the behaviours we see in others. It's an unconscious response, and there's nothing we can do about it. When someone smiles at us, our mirror neurons smile back at them. If we see someone being kind and helpful, we are more likely to be kind and helpful too; we've been 'primed' by our brains to be so. Mirror neurons are fired to make us feel empathy and compassion for others, even if we are only imagining how they are feeling. From the perspective of Love, when someone looks at us lovingly with affection, we are very likely to feel love and affection for them in return.

Of course, the same is true for negative behaviours and emotions. If someone looks very sad, depressed, unhappy, frustrated or angry, our mirror neurons also fire to reflect that. Mirror neurons are the start of what psychologists call, 'emotional contagion', whereby we pick up on and reflect back the emotions of the people around us. So be careful whom you spend your time with![5-6]

Oxytocin – the 'Love' Hormone
Closely connected with the vagus nerve and vagal tone, oxytocin is implicated in all sorts of human behaviours from holding hands and kissing, to the healing of wounds, from lactation and feeding infants to spending time with our pets. It's probably most famously known for being released at the point of, and just after, orgasm, where it encourages deep relaxation and trust between people and also promotes pair bonding, commitment and partner exclusivity.

In fact, oxytocin is released whenever we socialise with people, not just when we are with people we Love[7]. Oxytocin is released through any kind of social connectivity, which also physiologically triggers the release of serotonin within us, making social connectivity a biological 'reward'[8]. In addition, oxytocin is also released when we think kind or compassionate thoughts or are touched by others. This effect is magnified when we have a massage, and also when we give someone else a massage[9].

Interestingly, we also produce oxytocin when we're inspired. Perhaps that might go some way towards explaining why so many of us like motivational speakers or inspiring stories of courage or how people have overcome hardships to triumph. We find them uplifting precisely because the release of oxytocin gives us a physical, biological, 'lift' and makes us feel good. We think that it's hearing the story that makes us feel so elevated, and in a way it is. But it seems that it's our bodies' physiological response to hearing and internalising the story which is the uplifting factor[10].

Oxytocin is also fundamentally related to trust. It shapes and reshapes the neural circuitry of trust and the decision-making related to trust and generosity. In a ground-breaking study, inhaling synthetic oxytocin via a nasal spray made participants in a game of competitive/collaborative financial rewards and exchange both more trusting and more generous towards their playing partners, even after their partners had betrayed them[11].

Two of the implications of oxytocin in our daily lives are that firstly, we are more likely to trust people if we meet them in a social situation than we are to trust strangers. Secondly, we are more likely to trust a stranger if that stranger touches us in some way. Imagine someone we don't know who wants to sell us something. Now all of the random acts of touching your arm, shoulder, back or hand should be starting to make sense to you!

From a working perspective, those organizations which have a culture of shaking hands when colleagues meet, and the European equivalent for the ladies which is a kiss on both cheeks, are likely to engender greater trust, friendship and collaborative teamwork, than those organizations where colleagues simply say hello. I have noticed that multi-national organisations such as BP and Airbus for example are particularly professionally friendly, and this friendliness definitely does engender a feel-good environment and a sense of belonging.

From a Love and romance perspective, oxytocin makes strangers appear more attractive and boosts their sex appeal. This finding is true for both men and women. So, we will find strangers more attractive when we are already relaxed and in a social environment with our friends[12].

I mentioned the vagus nerve earlier. With the parasympathetic nervous system it works together to assist us to, 'rest and digest'. It seems that oxytocin also has a part to play here, as it's been found to promote gastric motility in the colon. Isn't it fascinating how all of these things work so efficiently and effectively together within us. It does suggest that there might be quite a lot that we could do to help ourselves with regard to IBS for example, which has been shown to have more severe symptoms when someone is stressed or upset. By deliberately doing some more of the activities which engage the vagus nerve and stimulate the release of oxytocin and increase vagal tone, potentially, many people could improve their physical health as well as their emotional well-being[13-14].

Atherosclerosis is the hardening of our arteries. In another medical study, oxytocin has been shown to protect the heart from atherosclerosis[15]. Married couples who are hostile towards one another have been shown to have higher levels of atherosclerosis than couples who are loving and kind towards each other. Once again, there appears to be a link between vagal tone and oxytocin[16].

Angiogenesis describes the growth of new blood vessels which is one of the critical processes in cellular wound repair. It's been shown that oxytocin can stimulate angiogenesis[17]. If oxytocin was for sale, it would be called a wonder-drug. The fantastic news for us is that very many things can stimulate its production within our bodies. We have an endless free supply!

There's a list later on in this chapter called 21 Ways to Increase Oxytocin Release and Vagal Tone. I expect that you're doing some of them already. If you want to increase your general health, wellbeing and happiness, do as many of them as you can, as often as you can!

The Science of Volunteering
In his book, The Healing Power of Doing Good, Allan Luks[18] describes a large scale study looking at the volunteering habits of more than 3,000 adult Americans where volunteering increased people's happiness and feelings of self- worth.]

In another study of more than 2,500 people, regular volunteering was found to improve six specific elements of people's wellbeing: general happiness, overall life satisfaction, self-esteem, personal agency, (i.e. the sense of control we feel that we have over our lives), general physical health and the absence of depression[19-21].

A 1999 study of nearly 2,000 elderly adults found that those people who could be labelled 'high volunteers', that's to say, they volunteered on a regular basis for two or more different organizations, had a mortality rate which was 44% lower than a control sample of similarly aged adults who didn't volunteer[22]. Similar results were found in a longitudinal study of more than 2,500 septuagenarians, where a 33% lower mortality rate was identified[23].

'Addicted' to Love
Falling in Love is so pleasurable partly because it stimulates the body to release feel-good chemicals within us such as dopamine and serotonin which affect the reward pathways of the brain. It was only relatively recently in the 1970's that scientists discovered that the body creates neuropeptides called endorphins which are natural opiates and which 'plug-in' to the brain via special receptors. We know that man-made chemical opiates such as cocaine, heroin and morphine utilize these same receptors. They not only give us a 'high', they are also highly addictive[24-25].

It turns out that we can also become addicted to the feel-good chemicals that we produce in our own bodies simply by thinking about certain things or people or through various behaviours. We can experience an endorphin induced high through exercise for example. Often called 'a runners' high', it means that some people effectively become 'addicted' to exercise. When injury or time pressures at work mean that they can't work out or run, they can become very edgy and unsettled, short-tempered or depressed. In fact, they often begin to behave like a drug addict who needs their next 'fix'.

Volunteers can also sometimes experience 'a helper's high' through a combination of dopamine, serotonin and oxytocin, which are released when we do an act of kindness for others. Sending or receiving a text message or email from someone we have just met and are romantically or sexually interested in triggers the same chemical responses in us. Even the anticipation of receiving an email or text can create an organic chemical high within us, as every cell in our body is effectively flooded with emotion.

This is why 'Falling in Love' with someone is so overwhelming; we become literally 'addicted' to them, and very quickly we can begin to crave contact with them. They can become all we think about, and if the relationship ends, we experience not just the normal grief at its loss, but also the chemical withdrawal symptoms similar to those which a drug addict experiences.

Of course the body is incredibly complex and nothing happens in isolation. So if you also add an element of danger into the mix such as the excitement of an affair, or even a slightly dangerous hobby, not only is the body flooded with oxytocin and opiate endorphins, it's also flooded with adrenaline and sometimes testosterone too. It's no wonder that 'Falling in Love' can sometimes make some people spiral out of control and behave in reckless, selfish or unusual ways.

The Science of Losing Love
If you remember the list in Chapter 1, The Characteristics of Losing Love, you will probably have realised that what we are really talking about is the neuropsychobiological science of both loss and the subsequent grief that we experience as a result of our loss. Let's unpick that a little as it's quite a mouthful! To really understand what's going on here at, what will be for all of us, the most difficult of times, we need to consider the neurological (brain), psychological (emotions and behaviours), and biological (what our body does), effects that happen within us, as a result of loss and grief.

How people respond to loss varies between individuals, however there are some common themes. Initially, the first thing that happens to us is that the initial shock of the loss will kick-start our sympathetic nervous system and we will most probably go into one of the fight/flight/fright modes which engages when we feel threatened and in danger. Our body will be flooded with adrenaline, noradrenaline and the stress hormone, cortisol, as we become primed for our immediate survival. We might go into a stage of complete shock, (fright), and not know which way to turn or what to do as we won't be able to think straight. We might simply want to flee, and run away from the situation and not think about it, because we can't or don't want to think about it, (flight), or we might become angry and try to argue our way out of the situation, often accompanied by refusals to believe or accept the situation, and denials that it's real, (fight).

We will all have a habitual mode which we usually go into when we experience major loss. But whichever mode we go into, our brains will be 'hijacked' by the flood of neurotransmitters and hormones, our pre-frontal cortex and neo-cortex will shut down. Remember, these are the home of our 'intelligence', our logic and higher executive thinking. Our brain will immediately go into what's called, 'Reptilian Mode', where the oldest and most primitive part of our brain takes over[26]. This state is neither pleasant nor comfortable, but deliberate practice can help us to manage it more effectively. This is something which airline pilots for example and jet fighter pilots are trained to do in case of an emergency, where calm, rational thinking is required and freezing, running away or fighting aren't appropriate options. (For more information, see 'Triune Brain Theory').

The vagus nerve engages to do the opposite of its 'rest and digest' function, and we will completely lose our appetite. We will also suffer from affected sleep patterns, either not being able to sleep at all, or disturbed, restless, wakeful sleep. Some people's hair will fall out, or, more unusually, it may appear to turn white or grey almost overnight. Some people, usually those who are already physically vulnerable in some way because of age or ill-health, may suffer heart failure or a stroke within weeks of experiencing a major loss of some kind.

There's no one timescale during which people experience this initial shock state. How long it lasts will depend on the individual, the nature of the loss, people's previous experiences etc. Everyone will eventually move out of this initial shock stage, however, it can take weeks, even months, particularly where the unexpected loss of a much-loved close family member or partner has occurred.

Once someone has moved through the initial stages of shock, disbelief and anger, often the next thing that happens is that people want to talk about the situation and their loss. They may repeat themselves, rerunning similar conversations with many different people as they try to comprehend what has happened. They are trying to understand and make sense of the loss, and often they are also looking to find some kind of meaning in it, if that's at all possible.

Because this second stage involves a focus on the person, pet, situation, relationship or job role that has been lost, many people often find much comfort in this stage. Engaging in Loving thoughts can be very healing as we already know. So it's very common for people to find themselves comforted as they are planning a funeral, for example, as throughout the planning and the activities involved in making it happen the Loved One who has passed is foremost in their mind. This can of course, keep some people 'stuck' at this stage, as they find it easy to access Loving thoughts and they can feel that their thinking brings them closer to their Loved One.

Emotional and physical healing won't take place at this second stage however if someone is angry and hostile, or depressed, or fearful of the future, as we know that all of these conditions will compromise the immune system. Eventually though, most people will reach the stage that psychologists and grief counsellors call, 'Acceptance'. This stage is the precursor to the most healing stage of loss which is 'Moving on'. It is only when someone has fully accepted the loss and is ready to move forward into their future positively, having let go of any pain, anger or grief, that true emotional and physical healing can occur.

We now know that this healing is facilitated by oxytocin, engaging the vagus nerve and strengthening our vagal tone. All of the things that I've described happen largely unconsciously and, for the most part, we have no control over them. Except that we do.

We now know that our thoughts profoundly affect our bodies at a cellular level, and that by changing our thoughts from anger, hurt and grief, to those of Love, loving and kindness, we can influence our body's auto-immune and inflammatory responses and change them from damaging us to healing us.

Once again, like a miracle which has been staring us in the face all along, but we simply couldn't see before, we can now understand that Love really IS the answer here, as it is in so many areas of our lives.

I apologise if you think that I'm being a little evangelical about it all, but as you will go on to read in Chapter 6, When Good Love Goes Bad, and also in the case studies in Chapter 9, you will come to understand, if you haven't already, that Love, loving and being loved, can have profound healing effects on our health emotionally, and on our health physically. The answers, and the cure, are within us. They have been there all along. It just needed the science to catch up with the psychologists and then for someone to knit together the relevant strands from science and psychology to make something tangible; a metaphorical cable-knit jumper if you like, which everyone can put on and wear if they want to feel better.

More on Vagal Tone
Earlier on in the chapter I introduced the idea of Vagal Tone, which put very simply, is the efficiency of your vagal nerve. Like a muscle, the more you deliberately use your vagal nerve positively, the higher your vagal tone will be. High vagal tone is very good for our health as lower vagal tone has been associated with inflammation, depression, anxiety, loneliness, negative moods, and an increased risk of heart attacks and strokes[27].

Stimulating the vagus nerve, which you can do by breathing, taking a few deep breaths with long exhales, or by thinking loving thoughts via Loving Kindness Meditation, has been associated with dramatic reductions in the body's inflammatory responses. This has major implications for the treatment of auto-immune conditions such as rheumatoid arthritis for example. A recent clinical trial demonstrated that pro-inflammatory cytokine production could be reduced in such patients by implanting a small device, called a neuromodulator, which stimulates the vagus nerve[28]. Stress and depression are also associated with increases in the production of pro-inflammatory cytokines as the immune system becomes compromised[29].

If we add this information about the health-giving benefits of high vagal tone to what we know about Loving Kindness Meditation being able to reduce physical feelings of pain, understanding the vagus nerve and how you can develop better vagal tone becomes simply one of the most important things that you will ever learn in your life. As in so many things, Love really is THE answer!

Amazingly, a number of studies have now shown that stimulation of the vagus nerve can prevent organ damage caused by severe infection. More than this, incredibly, where there has already been significant organ damage, stimulating the vagus nerve has actually been shown to be able to reverse some of the damage, even in tissue that doesn't usually regenerate[30].

There is also a link between inflammation and Alzheimer's disease. Potentially, therefore, by reducing inflammation we may be able to slow down its onset in vulnerable people and reduce its progression in those people who are already displaying Alzheimer's symptoms[31].

21 Ways to Increase Oxytocin Release and Vagal Tone
There are many ways to stimulate the release of oxytocin and also increase our vagal tone. As I said earlier, it seems that we've been biologically engineered to do them! There is more information in Chapter 5, Bringing More Love into Your Life, including a guide to doing a Loving Kindness Meditation.

1. Have Loving thoughts and feelings – towards others, ourselves, animals, the environment, God, the Universe et al.

2. Express positive emotions, (suppressing negative emotions increases the stress hormone cortisol).

3. Spend time socially, interacting with others, particularly where you are also having fun.

4. Spend time on hobbies and doing things that you enjoy so much that you experience a 'flow' state or, 'getting into the zone'.

5. Have a massage, or give a massage to someone else.

6. Do some deep breathing; deep breaths in, hold for a couple of seconds, then long, slow exhales out.

7. Find a story that inspires you, or a person who inspires you.

8. Spend some time in the company of someone you trust.

9. Watch a romantic comedy or feel-good movie, (e.g. Love Actually, Something's Gotta Give, French Kiss, 4 Weddings and a Funeral, Notting Hill, The Princess Bride, The Holiday and Passengers).

10. Do something kind.

11. Watch a favourite comedy show on TV.

12. Go to a Christmas pantomime or comedy club.

13. Go for a walk in the sunshine. This is magnified if you go for a walk in the countryside and if you take other family members, a much-loved dog, or in my case, ride a much-loved horse.

14. Get a pet and play with it, stroke it or watch it. Many people find fish tanks very relaxing, and I love watching my chickens in the garden. They always make me laugh; it's just like watching the film, Chicken Run.

15. Write a letter to a friend or a loved one telling them what it is that you love about them and/or explaining why you love them so much. Even if you never send it, the effect within you will be the same.

16. Do a shorter version of 15 by text, or just tell someone that you love them. Many people often tell their immediate family that they 'Love them' or that they 'Love them loads', but not that many people tell their friends that they Love them, although it's something that I often do.

17. Do a Loving Kindness Meditation or pray.

18. Make Love. Having sex will also release oxytocin, but to a lesser degree than 'Making Love' will. Making Love with a Tantric philosophy is particularly recommended, as everything a couple do within a Tantric philosophy is designed to deepen and strengthen the emotional attachment and bond between them. If you don't understand the differences between Making Love and simply 'having sex', it suggests that you need to learn more about understanding what Love really is. Fortunately, you're reading the right book to help you!

19. Kiss or hug someone, or hold hands.

20. Use your imagination to imagine doing any of the above! Remember, whilst your body might be able to tell the difference between actually doing something and imagining doing it, your neural pathways can't tell the difference, and your thoughts will be enough to make the body respond by engaging the vagus nerve and releasing oxytocin.

21. Listen to some beautiful music, or any music which you find to be uplifting.

Loving Relationships and Good Health
Having a loving, affectionate and supportive marriage is associated with having better quality health later on in life. Actually, I should really rewrite that, as it's not the marriage that is the important factor here, but rather the relationship itself, regardless of its legal or social status[32].

In stark contrast to those people who report being in a happy marriage, being in an unhappy marriage has been associated with significant increases in depression in more than one study[33-34].

Hostility and anger are some of the strongest predictors of high blood pressure and heart disease. Marital hostility has been shown to be particularly detrimental[35-38]. Hostility within marriage has been shown to promote the production of pro-inflammatory cykotines within the body as well as slowing down the rate of wound healing[39]. Cynicism and negative thinking linked with hostility is a particularly lethal combination for the heart[40].

It's not all doom and gloom though. Engagement of the vagus nerve and the production of oxytocin within a loving marital relationship has been shown to promote wound healing[41-42].

Intimacy is a stress buster! In a key study, intimacy, which the researchers defined as, 'physical affection such as holding hands, touching, hugging, kissing or having sexual intercourse', not only increases oxytocin and the other feel-good chemicals such as dopamine and seratonin, at the same time it's been shown to reduce the amount of cortisol present in our bodies due to daily work stresses[43].

Friendship is also cardio-protective. In a 1994 study of nearly 800 adults, (of approximately equal numbers of men and women), those people who reported the greatest amount of emotional support from their friends, were also found to have the lowest levels of stress hormones in their urine[44-45].

To increase your emotional well-being, get a pet!

Stroking a pet, especially stroking dogs, has been linked with improvements in the long-term survival of heart patients. Of course this finding may also be associated with increases in the cardio-vascular exercise required as a dog owner[46-47]. Some hospitals and nursing homes now regularly have 'petting dogs' to visit their clients because of the beneficial health benefits and happiness they can bring.

Another way to increase your emotional well-being, if you can't have a dog or another pet, is to get a plant! In a seminal study from the 1970's, elderly residents in a nursing home were given the responsibility of selecting a plant for their room and caring for that plant. (The control group were told that the plant's care was the responsibility of the nurse). The death rate of those residents with a plant to care for was 50% lower over the course of the study than that of the control group residents[48].

Reduced emotional expression in women, by which I mean women who don't express their feelings, but rather, internalise them without saying anything, has been linked to the rate of progression of breast cancer[49]. In this particular study, the researchers went even further to suggest that higher levels of oxytocin within women, (and therefore I would suggest, higher levels of vagal tone), may be a protective factor in slowing down the rate of progression within some breast cancers.

'Warm contact' is the term used by researchers to describe tactile and affectionate touching such as hand-holding, and also includes positive emotional support. Warm contact therefore can be either physical or emotional, or a combination of the two.

The giving and receiving of warm contact from a partner or loved one is associated with higher levels of oxytocin. Even the thought of receiving warm contact, that is the anticipation of receiving it, is enough to increase our oxytocin levels, while reducing blood pressure and the stress hormone cortisol[50-52].

In Summary
Love and loving, giving Love and being loved are all fantastically good for us in all sorts of ways. From preventative health to regenerative health, Love has a key part to play in helping to make us feel better.

I have come to believe that all 10 of the Love Types described in this book can heal and sustain us at a profound level, both emotionally and physically. Having just one of them in our lives is enough to increase vagal tone, reduce inflammation and stimulate the positive reward centers of the brain to release organic feel-good chemicals within us such as endorphins, dopamine, serotonin and oxytocin.

When we combine the Love Types and experience more than one kind of Love in our lives at the same time, the chemical effects in our bodies and the resulting positive physiological effects for our health, well-being and longevity are magnified.

Love really IS the Answer!

In the next chapter we will explore each of the 10 Love Types in more depth before going on to calculate, in Chapter 4, how much of each of the 10 types of Love you currently have in your life, compared to how much you would like to have.

Chapter 3

The 10 Types of Love

"Where there is love there is life"
Mahatma Gandhi, Indian civil rights leader.

This chapter explores the 10 different Types of Love. It will help you to understand each kind of Love more fully. I have included examples and short case studies for you on the less well known types because it's possible, even quite likely, that whilst you might recognise each kind of Love as familiar, as they are described to you here, you might not have given them very much thought before. Not many people spend much time differentiating between different kinds of Love. They feel it, they experience them, they grieve their loss, but they don't seem to really think about them very much.

The two most common questions which friends and colleagues asked me while I was writing this book for you, were, *"How do you work out what the 10 different Love Types are?"* and, *"How do they inter-relate with each other?"*

The first question is quite easy to answer and relates to vagal tome and oxytocin. The second one is much more complex, because the ways in which the Love Types correlate with each other may depend, in part, on each person. Scientifically, this probably isn't an ideal response, however, psychologically we know that there are always individual differences between people. So the ways that 'Love' is meaningful to you personally in your life, may be different to the ways that your friends or neighbours think about and experience it. More importantly, these differences in thinking about Love may well also be different to the ways in which your partner thinks about it. This book, then, if you would like it to, also offers you an opportunity for meaningful, insightful, profound and healing conversations with your loved ones around the subject of Love and what it means to each of you.

Identifying the 10 different Love Types was relatively easy and there were two parts to it. Firstly, I started by exploring the neurological and psychobiological effects that Love has on us. That is to say, the physical, emotional and neurological ways that Love influences what happens in our bodies when we experience it, and also importantly, what happens to us when we lose a particular kind of Love. If you are reading this book sequentially, you will just have read about passion, Love and loss in Chapters 1 and 2.

Secondly, I returned to the ancient Greeks. In modern Western language, we use the same word 'Love' for all of the different kinds of Love we experience in our lives without differentiating between them very much beyond Universal, Romantic, Familial and Friendship Love. The ancient Greeks recognised seven kinds of Love and had a different name for each one. So I then spent many hours considering how our modern life has changed over millennia and, as a result, may have evolved the ways in which we think about 'Love' and the things and the people we Love and feel passionately about.

In summary, the 10 types of Love with their Greek correlates are:

1. Universal Love	Agapé
2. Love 2.0	-
3. Romantic Love	Erotic
4. Familial Love	Storge
5. Friendship Love	Philia / Platonic
6. Playful Love	Ludus
7. Self-love	Philautia
8. Material Love	-
9. Love of Nature	-
10. Pragmatic Love	Pragma

Let's start exploring Love with one of the types that we are probably all familiar with; Universal, or Unconditional Love.

1. Universal Love

"Did I offer peace today? Did I bring a smile to someone's face?
Did I say words of healing? Did I let go of anger and resentment?
Did I forgive? Did I love? These are the real questions.
I must trust that the little bits of love that I sow now
will bear many fruits, here in this world and the life to come"
Henri Nouwen, Dutch Catholic Priest.

Universal Love is often conceived as the highest form of Love, and because it is so fundamental to our human existence, it seems that it has a number of different names. Pure Love is one and Unconditional Love or Unconditional Regard another. The Ancient Greeks had a word for Universal Love, it was Agapé and means, 'A Love for everyone'. Universal Love is a wholly selfless love.

Selfless love is the willing giving of Love to another without expectation of reciprocity or reward, and it is freely given even if there is an emotional, physical or financial cost to us. We expect our religious and spiritual leaders to display Universal Love and it's an inherent concept within both Buddhist philosophy and Christian doctrine, for example.

The concept of Universal Love is relatively easy to grasp. It is the unconditional regard for all people irrespective of age, creed, colour, disability, and despite of their behaviour towards us or anyone else. It is the compassionate and unconditional caring about someone simply because they are a human being. It is a wholeness of self and a passionate regard for all life, which may also extend to the unconditional passionate regard for the environment and planet, animals, flowers and trees for example.

"Love and compassion are necessities not luxuries.
Without them humanity cannot survive"
Dalai Lama, Spiritual Leader.

True Universal Love is problematic for many of us however, no matter how religiously or spiritually evolved we may think we are. To truly have Universal Love, we would have to love every person we passed on the street equally, certainly from the perspective of being willing to help them and support them if we possibly could. We would willingly, *"Forgive those who have trespassed against us"*, to quote Christianity's Lord's Prayer.

This would include criminals who had stolen from us or defaced our property, or terrorists who had murdered our friends and family simply because their religious beliefs differed from ours.

Therefore, true Universal Love is going to be aspirational for most people. However we can still experience elements of it, and as you read about and explore the other kinds of Love described here in this chapter, you will find yourself noticing that there are similarities and overlaps between Universal Love and some of the other kinds of Love. As I mentioned in Chapter 2, the Buddhist Loving Kindness Meditation, Christian prayer or a Reiki Universal Intentional Healing Meditation will all enable you to access the feelings of Universal Love.

The Characteristics of Universal Love

- Acceptance and forgiveness.
- Trust and respect.
- Kindness and compassion.
- Truth and honesty.
- Generosity of Spirit.
- Being prepared to pay the 'cost' if there is one.
- Being non-judgemental.
- Selflessly and willingly given.
- Benevolence and altruism.
- Unconditionally supportive.

> *"The greatest gift that you can give to others is the gift of unconditional love and acceptance"*
> Brian Tracy, Canadian American Public Speaker.

In original Confucian philosophy Universal Love is called 'Jen', which means 'benevolence'. It incorporates such ideas as human-heartedness, altruism, humanity and love. Later on, Mo Tzu taught Confucian Jen as Universal Love and 'Chen Ai' as a Love which doesn't make distinctions. In later neo-Taoist texts Jen refers to the universal extension of Love by which one becomes mystically united as one body with heaven and earth. This unification and the blurring of boundaries to reach a higher spiritual plane are both common goals and recurring themes within religious and spiritual teachings. This is because, as we now know, experiencing selfless, generous Love can change our physical, mental and emotional states.

Buddha also advocated Universal Love as an equaliser. That is, according to Buddhist philosophy, we shouldn't have a different kind of love for special things or Love one person over another. This is an impossible goal for many of us in the West as we love our family members more than strangers and we are often particularly attached to our personal possessions, (see 8. Material Love).

Within the ancient spiritual practice of Reiki, which originated in Japan, Universal life-force energy is channeled by the therapist or practitioner. Most usually involving the physical laying on of hands, Reiki can also be sent as intentional thoughts. This healing Reiki energy may be channeled to any situation, time or place, where the energy will be used for its highest purpose, whatever that may be, and whether we, as simple humans, are aware of it or not.

The Christian faith incorporates a similar form of Universal healing. We are familiar with it in the form of our personal prayers, which we offer up to God, and also in the laying on of hands to heal the sick. The Christian faith recognises that as incarnated human beings we will find true Universal Love difficult, as it is generous without question, accepting and forgiving without hope of reward, and devoid of personal ego. Christianity recognises that whilst God and Jesus have Universal Love for us, we humans can only aspire to be as loving.

Christian scripture writes about Universal Love in the Bible, in 1 Corinthians 13, and this rather beautiful passage is often read at Christian wedding ceremonies as a reminder to the couple who are about to marry of how they should love each other and their children in ways which reflects God's Love for them.

"⁴Love is patient, love is kind. It does not envy, it does not boast, it is not proud. ⁵It does not dishonour others. It is not self-seeking. It is not easily angered, it keeps no record of wrongs. ⁶Love does not delight in evil but rejoices with the truth. ⁷It always protects, always trusts, always hopes, always perseveres. ⁸Love never fails".
1 Corinthians, 13: 4-8.

Whilst I have said that Universal Love is aspirational for many of us, there are people who embody it. They are rare, and they are always inspirational. Here are two of them.

Sir David Nott, OBE. English Front-Line, War-Zone Surgeon.
BBC Radio 4, Desert Island Discs, 10th June 2016.
Sir David Nott is a very special man. He is a Crisis Front-Line Surgeon, operating in some of the most war-torn and dangerous places on earth. He's one of the UK's top Vascular Surgeons as well as being a General Surgeon who works in three different London hospitals so that he can keep his skills up-to-date. When asked if he cares who he operates on when he's working to save lives on the front-line, even if it's the enemy, his response was, *"I don't care who I operate on, ... we are all human beings".*

When asked if there's an emotional cost to him doing the work that he does, he replied, *"I do suffer, there's no doubt about it, ... sometimes it's almost psychotic post-traumatic stress".* It can sometimes take him more than 12 weeks to recover from what he's seen and from the ethical decisions that he's had to make. For example, if he operates on one soldier and uses all of the available blood, then there won't be any blood available to save any of the children or the other wounded who may be brought in later on in the day.

With his wife Ellie, he has set up The David Nott Foundation, which takes surgeons from all over the world and trains them to operate in war zones, as David himself has done, personally risking his own life and, against the odds, cheating death, for more than 20 years.

Jeff Kirby, Canadian Buddhist and Property Developer.
The Times Newspaper, Home section, 12th June, 2016, page 20.
Jeff Kirby is the Founder of The Flint Group, which re-develops run-down urban sites. He is using a project in Hastings as a test-bed community project for helping to rebuild lives and support neglected communities as he doesn't believe that simply handing out charity works.

"We call ourselves a compassionate enterprise, which is a completely different thing, … Governments simply need to encourage regeneration to create wealth and raise thousands of families out of poverty." Whilst waiting for planning permission on a building project in Hastings, Jeff decided, at his own cost, to renovate the site for the community into a temporary cultural hub called the OB Collective, using a team of ex-offenders and recovering drug addicts. *"We've given them access to our cash box and even the company's credit card and we haven't had a single issue. … If you give people self-respect, unconditional trust and total acceptance, it has to affect them, … and you wake up thinking you're doing a decent thing"*. His objective, he says, is, *"To detonate a nuclear bomb of goodness over the South Coast"*.

Consistent with his Buddhist philosophy, Jeff distributes 10% of the company's net profits amongst his team of staff and suppliers. He also gives the staff a big free breakfast, lends team members money, guarantees deposits for flats and pays for food and medical care where necessary. He donates a further 5% of company profits to charities in developing countries, *"To remind ourselves that we have a responsibility for the well-being of all living things"*.

Chapter 3: The 10 Types of Love

2. Love 2.0

*"Let us always meet each other with a smile,
for the smile is the beginning of love"*
Mother Teresa

Love 2.0 is a modern phenomenon. The ancient Greeks didn't recognise it as Love even though in essence it would have existed for them. However, after three thousand years our world has changed technologically in ways the ancient Greeks could never have imagined, and it is this which has facilitated the growth of a Love which has always been with us, connecting the lives of people.

Focusing on the body's physical and biological responses as we explored them in Chapter 2, it was the psychologist Dr Barbara Fredrickson who first used the term 'Love 2.0' in her 2013 book of the same name. She uses the term Love 2.0 to describe moments of positive connection in our lives. She calls them, *'Moments of positive resonance'*.

As you now know from reading Chapter 2, we are designed to Love. That's to say, our psychobiology is organised in such a way that when we experience a positive moment of connection, either with someone else, with an animal, or even in nature, our body responds by rewarding us with various organic chemicals such as serotonin to relax us and dopamine which triggers the reward centers of the brain so that we feel good. These two chemicals, along with oxytocin, combine to fill us full of feelings of positivity and general well-being.

*"Love is that micro-moment of connection that you share with
another living being. ...Within each moment of loving connection,
you become sincerely invested in this other person's well-being,
simply for his or her own sake"*
Barbara Fredrickson, Love 2.0, p.10

Moments of positive connection happen to us quite often, probably more frequently than we realise. We can also deliberately make them happen by a million small acts of kindness.

47

A smile at a stranger for example, sharing a joke at a supermarket checkout, giving up our seat on a bus or a tube to someone who would appreciate it, giving a cup of coffee or a sandwich to a homeless person, a look of understanding and support to a colleague whose clearly having a bad day, a positive text to a friend, an 'I love you' text to a partner or close family member. The opportunities to connect with others are endless.

The Characteristics of Love 2.0

- Selfless and kind.
- A 'feel-good' moment.
- Profoundly meaningful in that particular moment.
- Generous and willingly given.
- Unconditional regard in that moment.
- A willingness to 'pay the price' if there is one.
- Positive and memorable.

Facebook, Instagram and Twitter
Moments of positive resonance and connection, are, I believe, one of the reasons why Facebook and other instant social media systems have become so meaningful to people. Love 2.0 is one of the reasons why it's so easy to become 'addicted' to Facebook and social media and is also one of the reasons why people can suffer symptoms of withdrawal when such connections are taken from them or denied to them for some reason.

Facebook is a perfect way to experience Love 2.0, both to give it and to receive it. It enables us to connect positively with people from all over the world. That's people we actually know and also people we don't know in 'real life'.

Modern technology means that meeting someone in person isn't necessary to experience Love 2.0. People's positive messages to each other, particularly supportive messages after some kind of trauma, are often very moving and heartfelt and are perfect examples of positive connection and Love 2.0. I often find people's stories, and their photographs, to be completely inspirational.

3. Romantic Love

"I saw that you were perfect and so I loved you.
Then I saw that you were not perfect and I loved you even more"
Angelita Lim

There has been so much written about Romantic Love, or Eros as the ancient Greeks called it, that I almost don't know quite where to start. Romantic Love is the only type of Love that includes sexual love within it, and it's the origin for the words erotic and erotica with their implications for sexual arousal.

Romantic Love is always sexual to some degree, at least in its intention. In Medieval times there emerged an idea they called Courtly Love, which was a kind of 'pure' Romantic Love, often unrequited, whereby the object of a man's affections was adored from afar, almost as a way of attaining some kind of spiritual fulfilment.

"A love at once illicit and morally elevating, passionate and
disciplined, humiliating and exalting, human and transcendent"
Francis X. Newman, editor. The Meaning of Courtly Love, p. vii.

This makes absolute sense of course when we consider the ways that being 'In Love' with someone Romantically, which after all is at least partly based on sexual attraction, affects our thinking, our physiology, our emotional and our internal chemical, biological, states. Knights would perform various services for a Lady to emphasize their chivalry, bravery and nobility, and their love and devotion to the Lady, in ways not demeaned by the base, physical act of sexual intercourse.

So at one end of the scale of Romantic Love we have the pure, 'Being in Love', obsessional, fantasized, idealization in our heads of the object of our desires, and at the other end of the scale we have the physicality of Love; lustful, sexually gratifying and completely embodied in the physical attributes of the other person.

"You can't blame gravity for falling in love"
Sir Isaac Newton, English Mathematician.

So what is it then to be, 'in Love' with someone? Many of us will have experienced the difference then between being 'in Love' with someone Romantically, compared to 'loving' someone Romantically. There are differences in our thinking processes, our emotional responses, our physical states and in our psychobiology and neurology.

We explored this in Chapter 2, but let's just summarise the two states here because they are very different. A lot of damage can be done in a relationship by two people using the same words to say that they Love someone, and yet meaning very different things by it.

Romantic Love: Stages 1 and 2

Stage 1 I'm *'In Love'* with you (Honeymoon Period) Fantasy?	Stage 2 I *'Love'* You (Mature Love) Reality?
• I can't stop thinking about you, you are constantly on my mind. I obsess about you	• Your thoughts, your feelings, your physical and emotional well-being matters to me
• I'm terrified at the thought of losing you, your loss would kill me	• I know I will never lose you because I carry you around in my heart
• I can't bear the thought of you being with someone else and not with me	• I want you to be happy, even if it means that we're not together as a couple
• Love is blind - you have no faults that I can see, to me, you are perfect.	• I can see your faults and I accept them as a part of who you are.
• I can't bear to be parted from you, don't go	• I will see you again soon, take care of yourself

"Immature love says, 'I love you because I need you'.
Mature love says, 'I need you because I love you'"
Erich Fromm, German Psychologist.

"Thinking of you keeps me awake.
Dreaming of you keeps me asleep.
Being with you keeps me alive"
Anonymous.

It is often said in couples' counselling and relationship therapy that Stage 1 of a new Romantic relationship is the 'honeymoon period'; obsessive, physical, emotionally uplifting and energising but also exhausting with the ever-present fear of loss. It can last anything between 6 months and 2 years depending on circumstances. As the Love between a couple matures into Stage 2, it becomes deeper and more emotionally intimate, but less frequently physically intimate.

By understanding how Stage 1 resembles drug addiction within the neural pathways of the brain, it's easy to understand how some people can become 'addicted' to Stage 1 Romantic relationships. Such people will move on to someone new as soon as the relationship begins to slip into a Stage 2 state. Affairs are fueled by this, as for some people, they say that it's the only time they 'feel alive', and, like a narcotic, they begin to crave the high that it brings.

Rather than embracing the Stage 2 of 'Loving' each other, and using that as a way of deepening the communication and the bond between them, including a deepening sexual bond, many couples seem to 'drift apart'. Problem Pages and so-called Agony Aunt columns are full of letters from couples, (or at least one half of it), lamenting the loss of romance, lust, eroticism or physical intimacy.

They will often use phrases such as, *"We've become like brother and sister"*, (Familial Love), or, *"I still love them, but we're best friends not lovers"*, (Friendship Love), or even, *"I love them very much, but it's out of duty and loyalty for the family rather than any romantic or sexual feeling"*, (Pragmatic Love).

The Characteristics of Romantic Love

- There is a sexual element to it, or it may be completely sexually, lustfully, based.

- It's mentally obsessional, at least in its early stage and feels compulsive, as if we have no control over it.

- It's 'In Love With' initially, rather than 'Loving'.

- In Stage 1, it is blind to, overlooks or rationalises the faults and shortcomings of the person of our affections.

- There is an underlying and ever-present, fear of loss, especially in Stage 1.

- It usually matures, or transforms into another kind of Love which isn't quite as sexually oriented.

There are many thousands of books on the subject of Romantic Love. How to find it, how to keep it once you have found it, how to avoid it waning, what to do if it does fade etc. *"Do you love each other deeply but are not deeply in love"?* is one of the publicity straplines for the book, I love you but I'm not in love with you: Seven Steps to Saving Your Relationship, by Andrew Marshall.

Not everyone agrees with this sentiment. However, the underlying assumption here is that we should all somehow aspire to remain in a state of Romantic Love with our sexual partners, especially if we are married to them. After all, the sexual element of 'Making Love' is the only thing that separates Romantic Love from any of the other kinds of Love, and for some people, it is a sacred act.

4. Familial Love

> *"In family life, love is the oil that eases friction,*
> *the cement that binds closer together,*
> *the music that brings harmony"*
> Friedrich Nietzsche, German Philosopher.

This is the love that we have for close members of our family. It's passionate but not romantic, physically intimate but not sexually intimate. It incorporates maternal and paternal love, sisterly love and brotherly love. For some people, who are particularly close to other members of their family, their circle of Familial Love may also extend to include various aunts and uncles, cousins, nieces and nephews, grandparents and step-parents.

Of course it's also possible to feel Familial Love for those people who are so close to us as to become our 'family' even if we are not actually biologically related or related through marriage. We sometimes refer to people we love very deeply as being 'like family', and in the US and UK these passionate feelings often incorporate our pets. For some of us, our animals become an extension of our close family group.

Familial Love expands to include, encompass and absorb, new people into it. Having a child is probably one of the most familiar ways through which we experience this. Our Love expands very easily to include new members and it's a Love that endures over time even after a family member is lost to us. Familial Love signifies a bond which lasts a lifetime.

The ancient Greeks called Familial Love *'Storge'*, and it's the basis for the phrase, 'blood is thicker than water', meaning that there are usually stronger ties between blood-related family members than either non blood-related family members or simply good friends.

In fact, research supports this idea. In experiments with members of the general public, where they were asked to hold their hands in iced water for as long as they could bear to on behalf of someone else. The closer the blood tie was to the person, the longer they were able to hold their hands in the iced water[1].

In other words, we will endure physical discomfort or even pain for longer when we are doing it for Love. Fathers and mothers would endure greater discomfort if they believed that it would benefit their own children than they would for a nephew, niece or cousin. These results support the idea that, generally speaking, we Love our nephews and nieces more than we Love a stranger, and we Love our own children more than we Love our nephews and nieces.

We make 'sacrifices' for family. These might be sacrifices of our time, (many parents complain of being a taxi service to their teenage children, and yet we still do it!). Or we may find ourselves giving up other resources in order to save up for Christmas University fees. Most parents would risk their own lives, or even sacrifice them if they had to, to save the lives of their children.

We also forgive family. Like Universal Love, in many ways we Love our family unconditionally. At least for some people that statement will be true. For others, even Familial Love is conditional on 'good' behaviour, and if family members don't behave well, whatever that might mean, Love may be withheld, or something called Tough Love may take its place. (We are going to talk a bit more about Tough Love in Chapter 6, When Good Love Goes Bad).

The Characteristics of Familial Love

- Selfless and unconditional.

- Accepting and forgiving.

- It expands to absorb new family members with no loss of Love for the other family members already in the group.

- A lifetime bond and beyond, unbroken by time or bereavement.

- We will make 'sacrifices' for those we Love.

- Passionate but not Romantic.

- Physically intimate but not sexually intimate.

5. Friendship Love

"Your friends will know you better in the first minute you meet than your acquaintances will know you in a thousand years"
Richard Bach, American Author.

The ancient Greeks originally called this 'Philia' and it's now also known as Platonic Love. It signifies deep feelings of Love for someone who is not related to us, (Familial Love), and with whom we are not romantically or sexually involved, (Romantic Love). So it's passionate but non-sexual in nature.

One theory as to its origins is that the term developed to describe the deep feelings of commitment that brothers-in-arms had to each other when they had served together in battle. You will notice here the potential overlap with Familial Love, (in fact, we often use the terms, Brotherly or Sisterly Love), where really close friends, to whom we are committed and for whom we would make sacrifices, become as important to us as our lovers, (Romantic Love), and our close Family members are.

At its deepest, and arguably at its best, Friendship Love is the total acceptance of another person: knowing them intimately in an emotional sense; their lives, their loves, their hopes and dreams; their strengths and weaknesses, their joys and fears; their light and their darkness; knowing the very best and the very worst of them, and to Love them unconditionally anyway.

"A true friend is someone who lets you have total freedom to be yourself – and especially to feel. Or, not feel. Whatever you happen to be feeling at the moment is fine with them. That's what real love amounts to, letting a person be what he really is"
Jim Morrison, American Singer and Songwriter.

To be known, and within that, to be wholly accepted, is one of the most powerful kinds of Love there is, and is closely related to those elements of Universal Love we explored earlier in the chapter. The difference is that where Universal Love is general, for everyone, and for no-one in particular, here it's specific to one person. In other words, it's personal, and more than that, it's emotionally intimate.

Embodied Friendship Love, how we actually express our platonic Love, is shown by our loyalty and support. It's sharing our time, our possessions and our resources; it's being forgiving, making sacrifices, putting our friends' well-being above our own if necessary; protecting them and our friendship with them; and being there through both the good times and the bad.

"To love and be loved in return", can apply to a deep and intimate friendship as much as it can to a romantic partner, and for some people, their emotionally intimate friendships can be even more meaningful to them than their romantic or familial attachments.

All kinds of love can be powerful, and Friendship Love, like Familial Love and Romantic Love, is particularly powerful and passionate. Many people would sacrifice themselves to save their best friend.

The Characteristics of Friendship Love
* Generous and selfless.
* Prepared to make sacrifices and share resources.
* Emotionally and often physically intimate.
* Accepting and forgiving.
* Always believing the best of someone.
* Faithful and trusting.
* Honesty and truthfulness.
* Supportive and kind.
* Mutual commitment.
* Understanding and compassionate.

6. Playful Love

"This is the real secret of life,
to be completely engaged with what you are doing in the here and
now. And instead of calling it work, realise it is play"
Alan W. Watts, British Philosopher and Writer.

The ancient Greeks recognised the importance in our lives of play and being playful. They called Playful Love *'Ludus',* which isn't a Greek word, but rather, a Latin one meaning 'play'. Playfulness and Playful

Love can occur between friends, lovers, family members, work colleagues and even strangers. It can combine with other kinds of Love, and when it does so, our feelings of Loving become enhanced and even more powerful.

For example, when a family goes on holiday, perhaps with three generations of family members, (parents, grand-parents and children), we are already combining Familial Love with Playful Love. If the family then goes to the beach, skiing or to a specialist holiday camp set in the woods with log cabins, nature trails and bicycle tracks specifically designed for them to enjoy nature, then we can add Love of Nature to the mix as well.

Flirting combines Romantic Love with Playful Love. Remember though that Playful Love between non-romantically involved people is completely non-sexual. Comedy Clubs and dancing are becoming increasingly popular. Friends or strangers can laugh together or engage in other playful activities which can be shared between friends, family, lovers or strangers, sometimes combining Love 2.0 with Playful Love too, when people feel that they've, 'shared a moment', of meaningful interaction together.

Psychology reveals individual differences in people's desire for the amount of playfulness that they want in their lives. In part this can often be accounted for by increases in age. Once someone has grown up through their childhood years, many people consider 'playing' as childish. However, there are many adults who remain playful throughout their lives and they may even become more so once they have the 'excuse' of grandchildren to play with!

Perhaps our inherent desire for playfulness is why many people choose hobbies which allow them time to 'play', whether that's making jam, curtains and flower arranging, or gardening, abseiling, experimental cooking, climbing, flying, cycling, riding a horse or motorbike, sculpting animals in wood with a chainsaw or knitting! What one person might consider a dull pastime will be someone else's passion.

Loving to do something and finding it completely absorbing and fulfilling changes our brainwave patterns and our hormonal balance, flooding us with feel good endorphins and healing us on a cellular level. When we combine our passion for something with having fun, and especially where we can also include laughter and movement, or our friends, our healing is magnified.

When we combine Ludus with Eros, that's to say, when we are playful within a Romantic relationship, again, the feelings that we have will be magnified. Particularly in the initial stages of a romance when we are getting to know someone and exploring our compatibility with them, the combination of sexual attraction and playfulness can be explosive. There's a reason why in relationship counselling, it's said that, *"Couples who play together, stay together"*.

Recent 2016 research has highlighted the personal benefits of having fun at work. Being encouraged to 'play' with work colleagues in the form of spending time together at work-time social events has been shown to reduce worker's stress levels while increasing collaboration, creativity, productivity and general feelings of well-being[2].

 As you might expect though, there are differences between the generations, with older workers reporting that, overall, having fun at work is less important to them than it seems to be for younger generations who report that they enjoy things like 'Dress-down Fridays', dressing up for fund-raising charity days and fun-focused team-building events more than their older colleagues.

Teasing a friend links Playful and Friendship Love. Teasing someone you fancy links Romantic Love with Playful Love. In a great piece of recent research looking at 58 studies of over 19,000 people across 15 countries, friendly and playful banter at work between work colleagues has been shown to increase social and group cohesion, improve feelings of general health, well-being and happiness while also reducing feelings of stress and levels of burnout[3].

Knowing what we now know about Love, engaging the vagus nerve and its link to the parasympathetic nervous system, reduced blood pressure and healing, this makes perfect sense. Of course, we must include a caveat here as one person's playful banter can be perceived by another as harassment or bullying, but when it's done affectionately, Playful Love is one of the most powerful, supportive and healing kinds of Love there is.

There are also cultural differences within the workplace itself regarding of the amount of humour that may naturally be present within the working environment. Those places which are inherently stressful, such as the military, the fire service, the police, mountain rescue and other first responder organizations often use humour and a sense of playfulness as a psychologically 'protective factor' against the difficult situations within which people find themselves having to work. One of the reasons for this is that laughter has been shown to soothe distress in upsetting situations. So perhaps in some cases, laughter really is the best medicine after all[4]!

The Characteristics of Playful Love

- It combines very easily with some of the other Love Types.
- It's critical for some people, becoming very much a part of their personality and the way they live their life.
- It's characterized by having fun, a smile, or laughter.
- Some people become less playful as they get older.
- It's better shared with others.
- It can be experienced with friends, family, or colleagues, and is often done publicly with strangers! For example, a football match, pantomime, the circus, comedy theatre or in a cinema.

7.0 Self-Love

"Love yourself.
It is important to stay positive
because beauty comes from the inside out"
Jenn Proske, Canadian American Actress.

Over my years as a psychologist, as a specialist in personal development and relationships, and because of my PhD research into Authentic Leadership, I have come to understand that contrary to popular belief, the most important relationship that we will ever have in our lives isn't with our parents or primary carers. Although of course that's vitally important for all sorts of reasons, not least of which is that loving care, kindness and attention are crucial for healthy neurological brain development in infants.

I now believe that the most important relationship that we will ever have in our lives, is with OURSELVES.

Self-Love, along with Romantic Love, seems to be one of the areas of Love and Loving within which people experience the most doubts and difficulties. Certainly hundreds of books and articles a year are published on the subject – including this one! If we all had a healthy relationship with ourselves, based on accurate self-awareness, self-understanding and compassionate self-regard, there would be less need for many of the therapists, coaches, agony columns in newspapers and magazines and many of the books which swell the shelves under 'self-help', 'personal development' and 'well-being'.

The ancient Greeks recognised that Self-Love has its own internal scale. According to the ancient Greeks, Self-Love moves from Healthy Self-Love at one end of the scale to Unhealthy, (narcissistic) Self-Love at the other end of the scale, so for the ancient Greeks there were two parts to Self-Love. But I think they missed something. Perhaps within ancient Greek society it simply wasn't an issue, but I think that there are 3 parts to the scale.

I'm talking here about crippling self-doubts, a lack of self-esteem, poor self-image, a lack of confidence, or worse, the self-loathing that can lead to self-harming and addictive eating disorders such as anorexia or bulimia.

If you look at the Self-Love Summary Grid which follows, there seems to be only one kind of Healthy Self-Love, which sits in the middle, and yet there are two kinds of Unhealthy Self-Love; one at either end of the scale.

As you can see, true Narcissism, which is also commonly associated with both Psychopathy and Anti-Social Personality Disorder, which form what psychologists call, *'The Dark Triad'*, is much less common and is thought to affect around 10% of the general population. The actual figures have never been confirmed as they are difficult to research because people don't tell the truth! However, the % figures for the Dark Triad traits are thought to be significantly higher than 10% within senior leadership positions, and also, interestingly, significantly higher amongst men than women. (See the book *Divided by Gender, United by Chocolate: Differences in the Boardroom*, for the reasons why this is the case).

I personally think that these figures present a rather sad modern picture, and I only wish I could estimate that more than 45% of people have genuinely healthy levels of self-esteem and self-regard.

A note here: these % figures are representative of women. I estimate that there are probably 'better' healthy percentages for men, as men have the protective factor of testosterone which is known to increase feelings of self-confidence and self-worth.

Self-Love Summary Grid

Unhealthy (Lack of) Self-Love	(Ideal) Healthy Self-Love	Unhealthy (Too much) Self-Love
Up to 45% of women	Up to 45% of women	Up to 10% of women
Low self-confidence	Self-confidence	Over-confidence
Lack of self-esteem	Assertiveness	Narcissism
Martyrdom	Dignity	Extreme selfishness
Self-sacrifice	Self-respect	Aggression
Submissive	Self-regard	Bullying behaviours
Behaviours	Self-compassion	Unreliability
Self-harming	Self-acceptance	Inconsiderate
Often apologises	Self-forgiveness	Thoughtless
Very self-critical	Kindness to oneself	Unkindness
Bullied by others	Authenticity	Critical of others
	Emotional 'balance'	Sense of entitlement
		Never apologises

The Characteristics of Unhealthy Self-Love, (Not enough Self-Love)

- Feelings that your needs are less important than other people's.

- A lack of self-confidence, (sometimes severe).

- A lack of self-esteem, (sometimes severe).

- A lack of self-respect, (sometimes severe).

- Being overly critical of oneself and hard on oneself.

- Submissive behaviours.

- Self-harming behaviours, (not just knives or sharp instruments, but sometimes people self-harm with food or exercise, either to 'punish' themselves or as a coping mechanism, or as a strategy to help them feel more 'in control').

- Feelings of worthlessness.

- Thoughts that if someone likes you or fancies you, then there must be something wrong with them.

- May be bullied by others. This can also sometimes be linked to a 'victim' mentality.

The Characteristics of Healthy Self-Love, (Ideal Self-Love)

- Self-respect

- Self-regard.

- Kindness towards oneself.

- Acceptance and forgiveness towards oneself.

- Self-confidence.

- Dignity.

- Assertiveness, (where you feel that your needs are equally as important as those of other people).

- Authenticity, (as you have the confidence to be 'yourself' and you're not 'hiding' anything).

The Characteristics of Unhealthy Self-Love, (Too much Self-Love)

- Narcissism.

- Selfishness and always putting oneself first.

- A lack of compassion, empathy and concern for others.

- Unreliability.

- Lying and grandiose stories or ideas.

- Being thoughtless, inconsiderate or unkind towards others.

- A sense of entitlement or superiority.

- Possibly bullying or aggressive behaviours.

Where do you sit on the scale? Where would you like to sit, and how does your position on the scale relate to the scores you gave yourself on your Self-Love Audit? If you sit at the low end of the scale, what has happened to you to make you believe that that's where you deserve to be?

You see, I don't believe that anyone 'deserves' to lack self-confidence, Healthy Self-Love or self-esteem. Healthy Self-Love is what we would all want for our children, so let's become our own best friend and take steps to ensure that we have it for ourselves as well. Chapters 5, 6 and 7 will help you if that's what you need.

Self-Love, Self-Awareness and Self- Understanding
In more than 25 years of coaching and supporting others, I have come to believe that there's a special relationship between the interactions of self-awareness, self-understanding and Self-Love. Even though they may seem similar at first glance, they are not the same thing at all.
It is possible to have any one of them without the other two, or even two out of the three. But those people who are really happy and successful, and who really live their lives authentically, are those people who have made the effort to develop all three elements in their lives. More than that; they understand the connections between them.

Let me explain. Just because someone has self-awareness doesn't necessarily mean that they have self-understanding. They might be aware that they are doing something, (usually harmful to them or their relationships), but lack the understanding to know what's driving their behaviours. So self-understanding is critical. Only then, combined with self-acceptance and self-forgiveness, can someone, (usually with the help of a coach or therapist), begin to unpick what's going on for them to learn to understand their patterns.

The metaphor I use is that it's a bit like a woollen jumper which has holes in it. We need to unravel what's going on before we can reknit it back together again, this time, without the holes!

To give a very common example, someone can become aware that they always seem to attract the wrong kind of person into their lives romantically. This isn't specifically a female issue, guys do it too. Often they repeat a pattern of attraction and rejection which leaves them in a downward spiral. Once they have recognised this and how destructive it is for them in their search for healthy Romantic Love, they want to understand why it seems to keep happening to them and what they can do about it.

Of course, the specific reasons why this particular pattern of behaviour keeps occurring and reoccurring will be different for every person, although there are often common themes that emerge which have to do with feelings of self-worth and self-esteem and the ways that they were brought up by their parents or primary care- givers.

So, self-awareness is the first step; unpicking those patterns of behaviour, which involves developing more awareness of our own beliefs and values. Subsequently understanding how those ingredients have combined with the sum total of our life experience to create our unique personality and psychology is the second step.

You can't have self-understanding without first developing self-awareness around it. Developing your understanding of how other people are similar to or different from you may happen in parallel to your own self-understanding, but it's often something which occurs later. There's often just too much learning going on for us to also take on board what things may be like for others.

If I've made this process sound simple, I apologise. It isn't! It's complicated, messy, convoluted, repetitive and encased in all of our own special protective thoughts and behaviours, which we often mistakenly think will somehow keep us safe. Developing self-understanding can take years. In fact, it's a life-long journey as we constantly have new experiences, some of which can confuse us … until that is, we invest the time and effort to understand them.

The final ingredient is Healthy Self-Love, and it includes all of the characteristics of self-respect, of dignity, of feeling worthy and worthwhile, of kindness, generosity, trust, acceptance, compassion and forgiveness. Really liking the person we are and being our own best friend and being happy in our own company are also indicative of Healthy Self-Love.

Even with self-awareness and self-understanding, without the third element of Healthy Self-Love, no amount of self-awareness or self-understanding will stop the negative and critical self-talk which so many people, particularly women, beat themselves up with on a daily basis. If someone doesn't love themselves enough to believe that they are worth something and that their happiness matters, they will never be truly happy or truly successful, or truly at peace with themselves and the world. They will never be truly healed or truly whole.

Without Self-Love, they will never be motivated to travel along the often-difficult road of self-awareness and self-understanding to the destinations of self-acceptance and self-forgiveness that are always stopping and resting places along our journey.

A Note About Self-Compassion
Many people are compassionate towards themselves. As an element of Healthy Self-Love, compassion involves being kind to oneself, and may also include self-awareness and self-understanding. However, there are also many people who are not very kind to themselves, who are instead very harsh on themselves and self-critical. The reasons for this may be complex, and again will be tied up with someone's beliefs and values and childhood experiences.

However, a new study gives us some insight as to the personalities and some of the beliefs held by people who lack self-compassion. Those people who are harsher on themselves after making an error also tend to be more competitive than those who are more self-loving and self-forgiving. Being kind to themselves makes them feel less ambitious and less industrious. They believe that they are less likely to succeed if they are kind to themselves, i.e. they think that they are more likely to succeed if they are harsh on themselves. Interestingly, these same people reported feeling stronger and more responsible once they had been tough on themselves. So there's an inherent advantage for them in terms of displaying tough-love rather than self-love. They have a different way of loving themselves[5].

The sales and selling guru Zig Ziglar once said, *"When you are tough on yourself, life is going to be infinitely easier on you"*.

Personally, I think that life is tough enough already, but isn't it fascinating how people's words actually tell us what's going on for them inside their own heads and hearts and gives us clues as to their personality and character?

What we can take from this is that those people who are driven and competitive are more likely to display Tough-Love towards themselves and others, in the belief that ultimately, it will help them to win in life and make them more resilient and successful.

8. Material Love

"I love the practicality of a good car. You know what I mean?
And when I say 'practicality', I mean the complete practicality of a
Ferrari 458, a wonderfully fantastic every day car"
Hunter Hayes, American Musician.

This is quite an interesting Love Type and not one which perhaps many of us recognize. The ancient Greeks didn't have a word for Material Love, and it seems to me that it's a relatively modern phenomenon. It's the philosophy of thinking that our possessions form a part of the sense we have of our own identity[6].

I've included Material Love as a specific Love type because in modern Western society, we are often passionate about our possessions, and many of them bring us great joy. We do seem to 'Love' those things which 'belong' to us, and it's completely socially and culturally acceptable to do so. Whether we 'Love' our car, our home, our clothes, our shoes, our motorbike or bicycle, our artwork or anything else we might own, spending time with our possessions, cleaning them and caring for them and especially 'playing' with them, does elicit in us some of those characteristics of Loving which were listed in Chapter 1.

Material Love is rarely as strong as Familial Love or Romantic Love, however, we do feel passion for our most cherished possessions. Young children for example very often don't want to share their toys and will guard them jealously, only giving them up for someone they themselves Love and trust. Such is the psychobiology of Love.

Included in Material Love are those passions and interests which also form a part of our make-up, such as being passionate about history, education, architecture etc. I've included them here because whilst in themselves they are abstract concepts, they are all usually associated with physical things; often collections of things. Be that books, photographs, paintings or sculptures for example.

The Characteristics of Material Love
- They may be concrete things or abstract ideas.
- Protectiveness of our possessions.
- Spending time with them or doing them brings us joy or comfort.
- We feel passionately about them.
- Thinking about them and using them relaxes us.
- They are linked to our sense of identity about ourselves.

Buddhist and Zen philosophies counsel people against Material Love, warning us not to become too attached to personal possessions and to avoid valuing one object over another as doing so, and their subsequent loss, will lead to suffering.

9. Love of Nature

"If you truly love nature, you will find beauty everywhere"
Vincent Van Gogh, Dutch Artist

The Love of Nature is another kind of Love which the ancient Greeks didn't recognise. However, many people do Love spending time in nature and the natural environment and find it profoundly healing. After a tough day or a long working week, I know that crave nature, fresh air and the joy of being outdoors. When someone Loves the natural world and they don't have the opportunity to experience it, its absence can, in some people, lead to feeling low, or worse, feelings of depression. Perhaps this explains why, to lift depression, many doctors prescribe not just exercise, but outdoor exercise.

If your circumstances allow it, getting a dog which you need to walk twice a day, which will Love you with every heartbeat and which will very quickly become a Family member, is possibly one of the most healthy and Loving and healing things that you can do for yourself and your family. If you don't know it already, you will find that having a dog can combine Familial and Playful Love, a Love of Nature, Love 2.0 when you smile and wave and greet other dog lovers, and Friendship Love, with both your wonderful pet and the friends with whom you share them.

The emotional highs which some people experience when they are immersed in nature, such as a beautiful sunset, the Northern Lights, being by the sea, or the joy of canoeing up a river at dawn as the early morning mist bathes you in its cool embrace, all engage the vagus nerve and release oxytocin. This is magnified within us if we also experience feelings of awe or inspiration.

But the natural world isn't just sea and sunsets, it's every aspect of our natural world, from the smallest insect or the tiniest flower to the magnificence of the rain forest and the beauty of a frozen lake nestling in the Rocky Mountains. From Yellowstone Park in the USA with its volcanic geysers and amazing wildlife to the wild African plains of the Serengeti; the list of examples is endless and each of us will find joy in different things.

In a seminal study in 1984, researchers discovered that post-surgery hospital patients with bedside windows overlooking views of green trees in a Pennsylvanian hospital healed, on average, one day faster than other patients without a green view, needed significantly less pain medication and suffered fewer post-surgery complications[7].

The Characteristics of a Love of Nature
- A profound sense of 'feeling at home' in the natural world.
- Protectiveness of the environment.
- When nature, animals or the environment are hurt, we hurt.
- We carry images and feelings around with us about it.
- We crave nature when we're away from it for too long.
- Being with nature and within it is profoundly healing.
- We feel a small part of something much bigger than ourselves.

Sir David Attenborough, OBE.

"The natural world is the greatest source of excitement; the greatest source of visual beauty; the greatest source of intellectual interest. .. the greatest source of so much in life that makes life worth living"

One of the most famous advocates of the natural world and its importance is Sir David Attenborough. Now over 90 years of age, and with a broadcasting career spanning almost 70 years, he is recognized globally as the champion of our environment and he has inspired generations of children and adults alike with his ground-breaking documentaries. He is unswervingly passionate about every aspect of our natural world, from tiny insects and birds to giant giraffes and elephants. From extinct dinosaurs and their fossils to animals which are evolving in our lifetime. His very public passion for the natural world and for all life on Earth is a testament to the idea that a Love of Nature and the environment is real and should be included here.

Professor Brian Cox

"We are the cosmos made conscious
and life is the means by which the universe understands itself"

Advanced Fellow of Particle Physics at the University of Manchester, UK, and a researcher at CERN in Switzerland working on the ATLAS experiment at the Large Hadron Collider, Brian Cox has become the UK's face of physics. He has written and presented Secrets of the Universe on BBC television and his enthusiasm for understanding the science behind our physical reality knows no bounds.

His passion for the earth, the moon, the stars, the night sky and all of the elements within it is truly inspiring and has motivated many people, particularly children, to take up science subjects and use them to study our planet and the cosmos.

Obi, Wildlife Cameraman
Sometimes a job becomes more than just a job; it becomes a vocation. And sometimes a vocation becomes more than a dedicated career; it becomes our very identity, one which defines us and colours everything we do and all that we are. Very few of us however, outside the military, have to put our lives in danger when we do what we Love.

71

Charging bull elephants, raging rhinos, man-eating lions and the ever-present threat of poachers, all of which create a requirement for round-the-clock armed guard protection, is just another day at work for a wildlife cameraman. Obi has dedicated his life to making a difference to the animals on our planet and his passion is his desire to show us the real stories behind the headlines, even if that means risking or endangering his own life in the process.

In a world obsessed by football on a global scale, it saddens me enormously that so many people seem to care more about a ball being kicked around a piece of land than they do about the rape of our oceans or the imminent starvation and extinction of the world's majestic polar bears. Of course, as always, Love is The Answer, and ultimately, it's only the Love of Nature which will save our planet. Let's hope that enough people will learn to Love our world and the wildlife in it before it becomes too late.

The Ice-Warrior Project

The Arctic sea ice at the North Pole is melting. We know this is true, however we don't know exactly at what rate it's melting or the real depth of the Arctic sea ice which is left. The melting of the sea ice causes the temperature of our planet to rise dramatically. This in turn causes ice caps to melt and sea levels to rise significantly. Already some islands in the Pacific Ocean are drowning and ever-creeping sea levels are threatening both land animals and marine life in the coral reefs.

As the project Founder and the Leader of the expedition, Jim McNeill *is* the Ice Warrior. He has championed environmental issues for more than 25 years and has nearly died twice as a result; once by falling through a fissure in the sea ice and submerging himself chest-high in the icy, freezing water. Roped to an Arctic sledge called a pulk, he only just managed to drag himself out. Had he of died, all alone in the High Arctic, his body would never have been found.

This expedition, to the last unmapped Pole; '*the Northern Pole of Inaccessibility*', invites ordinary people to become involved and do extra-ordinary things.

As a citizen-science endeavour, schools, businesses and individuals are invited to follow the project and support it in whichever ways they can. Follow the teams as they study rare Arctic wolves and film our endangered Polar Bears. Track the depth of the Arctic sea ice with them on this epic adventure to the Northern Pole of Inaccessibility; one of the last places on earth not yet ever visited by mankind.

If you care about the environment and our planet, support the project at *www.ice-warrior.com* and help make a difference.

10. PragmaticLove

> *"Being deeply loved by someone gives you strength,*
> *while loving someone deeply gives you courage"*
> Lao Tzu

Pragmatic Love is recognised as being 'mature' Love, that is, a Love which has gone beyond the immature passions and 'madness' of the highly sexually charged Stage 1 Romantic Love. Pragmatic Love is a deep understanding between two people; usually two people who have been married or together for a long time. The ancient Greeks called Pragmatic Love, *'Pragma'* and it represents the kind of Love where an enduring and deep-seated commitment towards the relationship has replaced excitable Romantic passions.

The word Pragma isn't a Greek one, it's Latin and means *'Factual'* or *'What is done'*. Pragmatic Love involves showing patience and tolerance, being understanding, negotiating, compromising and making sacrifices for the benefit of the relationship over the longer term. Forgiveness, acceptance and forbearance are all evident here. Frustration and even anger may also be a part of the relationship at times, however these are endured and eventually overcome for the greater good and the ultimate benefit of the relationship and commitment towards the family group.

Often within a relationship where the focus is on Pragmatic Love, sexual passion and erotic, Romantic Love will be absent. Playful Love may also be a missing element.

However, platonic Friendship Love and Familial Love will often fill the gap, so that the amount of Love within the relationship is the same, and the commitment to the relationship is the same, it's just that the type of Love present within that relationship takes a different form.

The deep, loving commitment of Pragmatic Love is an enormous comfort to very many people. For some however, the elements of negotiation and sacrifice are not so willingly given. This can lead to sadness, frustration, resentment, even anger. Sometimes these are endured stoically, even though, as we know from Chapter 2, they are neither psychologically nor physiologically healthy, in either the short or longer terms.

Everyone's situation is different. However, I do think that in such circumstances, perhaps the most loving and healthy course of action would be to find a way of ending the relationship with Love, so that the loving relationship could continue in a different form; replacing Pragmatic Love with Friendship Love and Healthy Self-Love. I wish people could be less possessive, more courageous and with less fear of things like being alone, financial hardship and other forms of loss,

The German psychologist and psychoanalyst Eric Fromm referred to Pragmatic Love as, *'Standing in Love'* as compared with the Romantic idea of *'Falling in Love'*. Pragmatic Love endures in sickness and in health, despite any difficulties or problems, and has a focus is on giving Love and support rather than taking it. Romantic Love and Playful Love may be absent within a relationship where the predominant relationship strategy is a Pragmatic one. For many people this situation is quite acceptable, and in some cultures, many arranged marriages are built around it.

Many people however fundamentally miss the heady excitement of Romantic Stage 1 Love, and will end a Pragmatic relationship in the hope of beginning a new, more sexually exciting and passionate Romantic one, where the kind of Love which is experienced is a biochemically induced, obsessional, almost addictive one.

The Characteristics of Pragmatic Love
- Trusting and respectful.
- Deeply rooted understanding and acceptance.
- Commitment.
- Negotiation, compromise and sacrifice, willingly done.
- Giving and supportive.
- Patient and tolerant.
- Gratitude and gratefulness.

Crossing Boundaries
By now you will have realised that the 10 Types of Love can be fluid; they ebb and flow, grow and shrink, and can evolve, sometimes either combining with another Type, or changing from one Type to another, merging across boundaries. For example, you will probably know of a relationship where Romantic Love has become Familial, Friendship or Pragmatic Love.

In fact, it often does, which can become a problem for many couples, especially within a long-term, committed relationship, (frequently a marriage), where children have been born and raised. How often have we heard friends of ours lament that they have become *'like brother and sister'*, or *'like best friends'*.

As I've suggested before, the language we use on the outside is a reflection of what's going on for us on the inside. Here, the words are suggesting that whilst the Love still flourishes between the couple, the one unique thing that differentiates a Romantic partnership from any other kind of relationship is missing. It's sex and 'Making Love', which is the critical element here, something which many married women seem to forget. Faced with such rejection, is it any wonder that some husbands look elsewhere for the Love they need?

Thankfully however, for many couples, Making Love does include Romantic and Playful loving sex. The combination of these two kinds of loving are considered to be, (by many relationship specialists), the most healthy for a long-term relationship or marriage not just to survive, but to flourish and grow.

Where Romantic Love becomes Pragmatic Love, very often couples stop making Love lovingly and just, 'have sex'. It's often perfunctory, quick, better for one person than the other, and often leads to frustration, or worse, infidelity, as one or both partners seek to supplement their Pragmatic Love for each other with a Playful or Romantic friendship with someone else.

Happily, in the opposite direction, Pragmatic, Playful or Friendship Love can also sometimes transform to become Romantic Love. Arranged marriages are common in some cultures, and these can sometimes transform over time from a Pragmatic, practical arrangement into one where 'True Love', in other words, what we associate as Stage 2, Romantic Love, begins to flourish between two people who, after all, are already in a committed partnership with each other.

Touch and text flirting, one-night stands, booty-calls, 'Friends with Benefits' and the like, whilst technically being Romantic in nature because of their sexual element, also fall within the broad spectrum of Playful Love. They can be enjoyable and fun and they are often emotionally as well as sexually intimate. Sometimes they can cross the boundaries into Romantic Love, although this is rare.

A word of warning here. Because in such situations we feel, 'loved', these things can quite easily become addictive, even (self) abusive, especially for young men and women who crave Love and physical or emotional intimacy. Or, we can 'fall in Love' and develop feelings which are not reciprocated, which ultimately hurts us.

You especially need to avoid such behaviours if you lack self-confidence or self-esteem. You may think that any attention is better than no attention and you may mistake the Playful attention for loving Romantic interest. Hundreds of hours of counselling clients has shown me, time and time again, that before you can have a healthy relationship with someone else, you really must have a healthy relationship with yourself.

If you find yourself in such a relationship, whatever age you are, there are three important things to remember.

Firstly, it's important to be self-aware enough to understand your motivations in the first place and also to understand the impact that such behaviours are having on your life.

Secondly, if you can, have an open and honest conversation with your partner about the kind of relationship you each want and the roles that the different kinds of Love might play in that. Wanting different things can often be confusing, or worse, hurtful and damaging.

Finally, make sure that you always stay on the healthy side of Self-Love and end things if the relationship begins to cause you pain or distress.

In summary once again, the 10 Love Types are:

1. Universal Love
2. Love 2.0
3. Romantic Love
4. Familial Love
5. Friendship Love
6. Playful Love
7. Self-Love
8. Material Love
9. Love of Nature
10. Pragmatic Love

In the next chapter you will have the opportunity to complete your Love Life Audit and to identify how much of each Love Type you have in your life, and, perhaps more importantly, how much of each Love Type you would ideally like to have.

Chapter 4

Love Life Audit: How Much Love do you have in your Life?

"Love many things, for therein lies the true strength,
... and what is done in love is done well"
Vincent Van Gogh, Dutch Artist

Now that you've read Chapters 2 and 3, you will be much more aware of the different kinds of Love which surround us. You will also have a much greater understanding of how bringing them into your life has beneficial effects for your happiness and health, and the happiness and health of the people around you.

As a result of this new awareness and appreciation, you will probably already have begun to think about how much of each of the different kinds of Love you currently have in your life. This may have been an unconscious process for you or you might have thought about it more deliberately. This next question then, may be a real game changer for you.

How much more or how much less of each of the 10 types of Love do you want in your ideal life compared to how much you currently have in your day-to-day reality? This question may be driven by a mild curiosity. Or, it may be a much more important question for you, the answer to which may change some of your future thinking and some of the decisions and actions you will take. There may be some kinds of Love you would like more of, and there may be some kinds of Love that you would prefer to have less of in your ideal world.

Your Love Life Audit is unique to you; there is no 'correct' profile. It's a reflection of your circumstances and the people currently have in your life. If you were to complete your Love Audit again in a year's time, you might find that the picture that emerges will be different from what's happening for you in your life right now

Before you complete your Love Life Audit let's review each of the Love types to remind you of their key elements and characteristics.

1. **Universal Love.** The generosity of spirit to Love all people equally, accepting them and forgiving them unconditionally.

2. **Love 2.0.** Moments of positive connection and resonance between you and someone else, or an animal.

3. **Romantic Love.** Physical, sexual attraction and loving feelings towards someone, which are more than lust.

4. **Familial Love.** The love between family members, which is usually stronger the closer the blood-line connection.

5. **Friendship Love.** Non-sexual love between two people who are not familiarly related.

6. **Playful Love.** Playing and experiencing fun or laughter, alone, with someone, something or with an animal.

7. **Self-Love.** Healthy self-regard, self-understanding, compassion, kindness and respect towards yourself.

8. **Material Love.** Passion for possessions or material things, which bring you joy when you are around them.

9. **Pragmatic Love.** Practical, mature and enduring Love within a long-term, committed relationship.

10. **Love of Nature.** A passion for, and commitment to, the environment and the natural world.

To Complete Your Love Life Audit
Using a scale of 1 – 10, where

1 – 3 is Quite Low,
4 – 7 is Moderate and
8 – 10 is Quite High

Complete the grid for your Love Life Audit which follows using the following 4 steps:

Steps 1-4

Step 1 - Identify your score for the amount of Love for each of the 10 types that you currently have in your life. Use your intuition and you will find that you will know what your score is.

Step 2 - Estimate what your ideal score would be for each type. Again, allow your intuition to guide you.

Step 3 - Calculate the gap between your two scores for each Love Type on each of the horizontal lines. You may have a positive gap, a negative gap, or no gap at all where your two scores are equal.

Step 4 – Add up your overall summary scores.

In an ideal world, your current and ideal scores will be the same, meaning that your 'gap' for each Love Type will be zero. If this is the case then you are very fortunate. Most people will calculate either a positive or a negative score against at least some of the 10 Love Types. I know that I did!

Remember that these are your personal scores, no-one else's! And there are no right or wrong estimations. We will be spending some time exploring what you might like to do about any gaps you have identified a bit later on in this chapter.

In Chapter 5 we will be looking specifically at how you can bring more of each of the Love types into your life should you choose to do so.

Love Life Audit

	Love Type	Current Score	Ideal Score	Gap +/-
1	Universal Love			
2	Love 2.0			
3	Romantic Love			
4	Familial Love			
5	Friendship Love			
6	Playful Love			
7	Self-Love			
8	Material Love			
9	Love of Nature			
10	Pragmatic Love			
	Summary Totals			

Key

1 – 3	Quite Low
4 – 7	Moderate
8 – 10	Quite High

In the process of writing this book, and this chapter in particular, I've completed a Love Life Audit three times over a two year period. Every time I've completed it my scores have changed in some areas, leading me to realise and more fully understand that, whilst I'm not lacking in Love overall, there are some specific areas where I would actually like to bring more Love into my life!

What thoughts immediately come to mind now that you have completed your own Love Life Audit? Do you feel that your Love Life is in balance and on track, or are there some changes in certain areas that you would like to make?

You may find that you have a number of thoughts surrounding your Love Audit, so find yourself a pen and some paper and I would suggest that you complete the following process, as it will assist you in getting your thoughts in order. It may take you 20-30 minutes, so make yourself a drink if you want one and, find somewhere comfortable to sit where you can think and write easily, ideally in a place and at a time where you won't be disturbed.

Completing this exercise could be some of the most important 30 minutes of your life. It will really allow you to focus on your whole Love Life, holistically, in every area, not just in terms of your Romantic Love Life, which after all, is what most people think about if the phrase 'Love Life' is ever mentioned! You will know by now that there is so much more to our Love lives than just that.

Before you complete this next Review exercise, if you would like to read an example of a completed Love Life Audit and Review, I have included one for you a little bit further on in the chapter. It's actually my own Love Life Audit and Review, which I completed to make sure that the process will work for you.

If you don't want to use the Audit Grid in the book, you can print off a blank copy of it from the Resources page on my website at *www.cognitivefitness.co.uk*

Love Life Audit Review

Step 1 – Using your Audit grid, go through each Love Type quickly and where you have a gap of 3 or more, (either positively or negatively), put a little star beside it. This will assist you later when we begin to look for any patterns you may have in your profile.

Step 2 – This is probably going to take some time, and you may have some personal insights as you work each line through. Jot your insights down and capture your thoughts because they will be important. Go through each Love Type in turn and write down what you think the reasons are for any gaps you might have. This will give you clues as to what you're not entirely happy about in your Love Life and, therefore, what you might want to consider paying more attention to, and possibly changing in the future.

Step 3 – This is where we are going to look for any patterns in your Love Life Audit. It's quite likely that if you have scored yourself -3 or more in your gaps, that these may somehow be related to at least one other Love Type. Recognising any patterns in your profile gives you more opportunity to do something about them, as by making any changes in one area, you will influence the others and make an impact on those too.

Step 4 – Using those thoughts you jotted down in step 2, and going through each Love Type separately again, write down some specific things that you could do, or even better, would like to do, to reduce the size of any gaps you might have. If you can't think of anything, we will be exploring this a bit more in Chapter 5.

Author's Note

Exercises like these can sometimes be easier to do if they are facilitated in a workshop environment, or if you are doing the exercise with someone else. As we don't have those opportunities here I have included an example for you over the next few pages.

Love Life Audit – Fiona Beddoes-Jones, 5th December 2016.

	Love Type	Current score	Ideal score	Gap +/-
1	Universal Love	6	8	-2
2	Love 2.0	6	8	-2
3	Romantic Love	3	8	-5*
4	Familial Love	7	7	0
5	Friendship Love	7	7	0
6	Playful Love	5	8	-3*
7	Self-Love	4	9	-5*
8	Material Love	6	7	-1
9	Love of Nature	5	8	-3*
10	Pragmatic Love	3	3	0
	Summary Totals			-21

Key

1 – 3	Quite Low
4 – 7	Moderate
8 – 10	Quite High

Step 1 – Complete, as you can see in the example above.

Step 2 – So that it's easier for you to read, I'm going to write a short paragraph for each Love Type.

Universal Love – A score of 6 for my life as it currently is puts me in the mid-range, that's to say, I would estimate that I probably have about as much Universal Love for mankind and humanity as most people do. I'm fairly liberal and tolerant, and I am our community's Parish Church Warden, which means that it's my role in the community to be loving and kind and generous and pleasant to people, (which I would always be anyway, even if it wasn't my specific role to be so). But I've thought about it and I would like to be more Universally Loving.

I'm sure that there's more that I could do, probably from a spiritual, and possibly from a community perspective. I would like to be thought of as a lovely person, but I think that I have a way to go before everyone thinks of me like that, if it's even possible. So my gap score of -2 reflects my aspirations to be kinder when I have the opportunity to be so, and to be more spiritually evolved.

Maybe writing this book is a part of that, a part of a, 'Generosity of Spirit', that I can aspire to. I don't know. I will have to give it some more thought.

Love 2.0 – I always try to brighten up people's days. I'm always very positive and upbeat with a smile and a kind word for everyone, whether that's in the post office, in the supermarket check-out queue or on the phone. I often tell little old ladies that they look beautiful, and I often pay the bridge toll for the car behind me, even though they are a stranger. But I still feel that I could do more, and I would like to do more.

Again, perhaps my ideal score of 8 is aspirational rather than realistic, but I would still like to be, 'My Best Self', more of the time. It makes the other person feel good and it makes me feel good, so I'm going to make a concerted effort to, 'spread the Love', and do more of Love 2.0, just because I can, and because it's nice to be nice.

Romantic Love – Ouch! This is a big one for me. I've just come out of a 22 year marriage, which I ended for reasons I won't bore you with. One of the reasons it took so long to end the marriage was that, for our daughter's sake, I didn't want to metaphorically tear the heart out of my family, and so I did my very best to be loving and supportive and kind towards my ex-husband so that we could, if at all possible, remain on friendly terms.

After all, one day our lovely daughter will most likely marry, and I don't want her day to be spoilt by having parents who can't bear to be in the same room as each other. How is that loving? It isn't, therefore I won't go there, even though there is an emotional cost to me to maintaining and encouraging continued friendly and loving communications with my ex-husband. So I have a gap score of -5, which reflects my desire to meet someone and fall madly and passionately, Romantically, 'in Love' with them, and experience that heady mix of hormones, emotions and elation described in Chapter 2.

Familial Love – I'm quite happy with this one. With my 3 siblings and their families, we're quite a close family, more so since our lovely mother suffered a catastrophic stroke some 6 months ago. We didn't lose her, thank goodness, but she's virtually completely paralyzed and she will never speak again. She's in the most wonderful nursing home and if anything, the tragedy has brought us closer together. So no gap here. Maybe the new man in my life will have some children of his own so my daughter and I will get to expand our immediate family and Love some more incredible people. But for the time being, all is well just as it is.

Friendship Love – I'm really lucky, I have some great friends, both male and female, and it's not at all unusual for a phone call, text conversation or email to end with the words, *"Love you loads"* or *"I Love you very much"*, from each of us. I think I'm a good friend. I certainly always try to be 100% supportive and to be available for my friends through the good times and any bad ones. I know a lot of people, and I have a lot of acquaintances through my work, in fact I'm always meeting new people. Sometimes we both get lucky and the spark of shared interests and values becomes a rock-solid friendship, which will last a lifetime. So no gaps here either.

Playful Love - I just love to be playful, mess around and have fun. I love Christmas Pantomime, comedy shows, baking with children, flower-arranging, riding my horse, singing in the choir, a day out to a giant adventure playground and throwing a ball for our dog. There are so many opportunities to play around and have fun as an adult and I love them all. I'm even playing a part in a comedy sketch show in a comedy review next year!

I've always had an enormous capacity for fun and my sense of humour is a big part of my personality. I've given myself a -3 here though so it's definitely an issue for me as I'm not having anywhere near as much fun as I'd like to have. Because of a serious knee injury a month ago, I can't dance at the moment, nor can I ride my horse or get out and walk the dog in the countryside. I'm so busy writing this book and with all of my other work projects that time for myself pursuing my own hobbies is very scarce at the moment, so I really would like to redress the balance.

Self-Love – Oh dear, another ouch! moment for me here with a gap score of -5! With a current score of 4 it's not that I don't love and respect myself, I do …. just obviously not enough! My current and gap scores were a bit of a shock to me to be honest. I don't think I realised quite just how bad things had got here in terms of looking after and nurturing myself.

I've become so used to making sure that everyone else is ok, especially because of the divorce, that I never put myself first, possibly because I would never want to be selfish in anyway.

Unfortunately, the net result is that I haven't looked after myself, and now I really need to. Starting HRT has made me go up two dress sizes, and pressures of work have meant that I simply haven't scheduled in any 'me' time, whether that's for a hobby activity I enjoy and which relaxes and nurtures me, or eating and exercising properly.

I'm limited to the exercise I can do because of my knee, which is currently twice the size of the one on my other leg, but there's no excuse to be slack on my nutrition just because I'm busy!

My score of 9 for my Ideal might seem a bit high, but this is Healthy Self-Love remember, not selfish, narcissistic Self-Love, and I really believe that we need to Love and nurture ourselves, after all, Love Is The Answer!

Let's think about it for a moment, would we tell our children or our best friend that they need to nurture or care for themselves less? – no, of course we wouldn't. So I'm going to stick with my 9 and hope that I can shift my actual score up at least a few notches over the coming months!

Material Love – I have some beautiful things, things that give me complete pleasure and joy when I look at them or use them. Like my bronze cutlery set of knives and forks with their red rosewood handles which almost take my breath away with their beauty and craftsmanship. But I don't always stop and take a moment to appreciate them, and my house is a little untidy at times so my beautiful things are not always displayed to best advantage.

In fact some of my most precious and gorgeous things are kept wrapped up in drawers or cupboards. This keeps them safe, but means that I don't get to enjoy them as much as I could. So my -1 score here reflects that. By being mindful of these things, there's more I can do here to bring more joy and Love into my life, and I would like that.

Love of Nature – Another wake-up call for me here. I live in the countryside because I love it. Anything more than a rural village location would be too suburban and built-up for me. So I live in a small hamlet surrounded by green fields filled with sheep and cows and brown ploughed fields, over which red kites and buzzards hunt for food on the warm up-winds. I hadn't realised quite how much not being able to walk our dog or ride my horse in the beautiful countryside has been affecting me.

I have a phone and a computer full of the most beautiful pictures of nature and the natural world, but I can't get out into it. Something needs to change. I find nature of all kinds to be completely joyful and intensely healing, and so this is one area where I definitely want the gap to be zero!

Pragmatic Love – I think that maybe I might have over-reacted a little here! My gap score is zero, which is great, but my Actual and Ideal scores are both a 3, which may be a little on the low side. The last time I completed my Life Love Audit, my Actual score was a 9 and my Ideal score was a 5, so there's been a big shift for me here.

The previous time I completed my Audit I was right in the middle of the divorce, I had my Decree Nisi but not the Decree Absolute and I was very frustrated as my ex-husband dragged his heels and played an unintentional game of 'head in the sand'! I had to bite my tongue on many occasions, so I really was having to be practical and pragmatic and make emotional sacrifices just to get through every day. I don't ever want to have to go through that again, and whilst I absolutely recognize the value of long-term, committed and deep-felt enduring Love, at the moment I want to experience the dizzying heights of Romantic Love first!

Phew! An interesting exercise, and if I'm honest, not one which was always completely comfortable, especially as I've effectively shared some of my innermost thoughts and feelings with the World!

So now let's complete Step 3 and explore any patterns that I may have in my profile. You might already have spotted a few as you've been reading through. They're not all things that I want to change, I'm very happy with some of them!

Pattern 1 - Universal Love and Love 2.0 are both -2 and they seem to go together for me, so I think that by doing more of one I will impact and increase the other, so I'm going to think about what I can do here for both of them.

Pattern 2 – Family and Friendship Love are both all 7's with a gap of zero which is great. I'm very happy with these.

Pattern 3 – Playful, Nature and Self Love all seem to be connected for me. By spending a bit more time having fun, and also getting out into nature and the beautiful world around us, I will be nurturing myself, so this is definitely a pattern I can impact on.

Pattern 4 – Romantic Love. This seems to be a stand-alone area of my profile rather than a pattern connecting Love Types per se. Once I've met someone special I'm sure that Romantic Love will connect with Playful Love, Healthy Self-Love and eventually Family Love.

I'm emotionally open to meeting someone special, but whether I do or not will probably be an accident of fate, and of course I can't have a Romantic relationship with someone until I've met them! So I'm just going to put this one on the back-burner for now and get on with the rest of my life. It will happen when it's meant to happen. I'm quite happy to be relaxed about it and let life happen around me and to me, enjoying as much of it as I can. The Purpose of Life is to Live remember!

Step 4 – I'm sure that you've read quite enough about me! This book isn't about me and my life, it's about you and yours, so I'm just going to suggest that you have a look at Chapter 5 and select some things from the lists under each type when you get to Step 4 or your own Love Life Audit Review, adding some things of your own too of course!

So that's it for this chapter. Now's the time for you to complete your own Love Life Audit, if you haven't already done so. I hope you find it as insightful and useful as I found completing mine to be.

Chapter 5

Bringing More Love into Your Life

"Kindness in words creates confidence.
Kindness in thinking creates profoundness.
Kindness in giving creates Love"
Lao Tzu

Having just completed your Love Life Audit, there may be some areas of your life that you would like to bring more Love into. So this chapter is full of ideas on ways in which you can do that. For simplicity, I've divided them by Love Type, although you will find that some of the suggestions cross boundaries and impact on, or involve, one or more of the other kinds of Love. Of course, this makes them even more powerful and magnifies the Loving impact that they will have in your life. Just like the list in Chapter 2, all of these things will increase your vagal tone and release oxytocin.

There are a million and one loving gestures you could do, some of them will be uniquely personal to you and to the relationships that you have. Some of them will cost nothing, and some of them may involve a financial outlay. Where this is the case in the suggestions I have included here, I have tried to keep the costs small. Of course, if you can afford it, and you would like to hire a plane to write *'I Love You'* in smoke above your house, then feel free!

1. Universal Love

"Keep love in your heart.
A life without it is like a sunless garden when the flowers are dead"
Oscar Wilde, English Writer and Poet.

- Volunteer for a cause you believe in, something that makes a difference somehow to the lives of others, even if you will never meet them and can only support them from afar.

- Say a prayer, or do a Loving Kindness Meditation, and include people whom you don't know in person but who need love and support. For example, all those who are sick, refugees who have no place to call home, the recently bereaved and people living rough on the streets who don't have enough to eat, the very poor and the lonely.

- Forgive someone who has wronged you. This will usually be a stranger, in my case the thief who broke into my car stealing the bag of gifts I had just bought for my friends and family. They were not on display and I very rarely leave anything in my car, so I guess I was just unlucky. But from the perspective of Universal Love, maybe he needed them, or the money he could get for them, more than I did.

- Contact *DKMS.org.uk* and register online to take a simple cheek swab by post to see if you're a match for a leukemia sufferer who might otherwise die without your help. Blood cancer can be curable if a matching donor can be found. Although there are already 27 million donors within the UK, many people still cannot find a suitable match. Becoming a blood stem cell donor could save someone's life.

- Willingly do something kind for someone, something which involves an investment of your time, and goes beyond 'a moment' of positive resonance, (which is Love 2.0). This may be a stranger, someone in your community or a friend of a friend. Note that If they are family, technically this gift of your time becomes Familial Love, or if they are a friend, then it becomes Friendship Love.

Love 2.0

"Carry out a random act of kindness, with no expectation of reward,
… one day someone might do the same for you"
HRH Princess Diana Spencer

- Do something nice for a stranger you've just met or even someone you don't know and will never meet, such as paying the road or bridge toll for the car behind you.

- Buy an extra sandwich, bottle of water and piece of fruit when you organise your own lunch. Give these to a homeless person, a beggar, or someone selling 'The Big Issue'. (In the UK, this is a weekly magazine which homeless people sell on the streets to earn money).

- Help an elderly or less-able person with something useful to them. For example, carrying their shopping, reach something for them, which is too high in a supermarket for them to get it for themselves.

- Say something nice to a stranger in a queue, which will make them feel better or give them a 'lift' in some way.

- Make a sign saying 'Free Hugs'. Attach it to yourself and wear it for an hour in a busy shopping centre or on a busy street. Hug everyone who wants one. Do remember to smile and look friendly though ….. if someone doesn't see you smiling and being approachable, they may become uncomfortable around you, which is the exact opposite of your intention! Remember your mirror neurons!

2. Romantic Love

"It was not into my ear you whispered, but into my heart.
It was not my lips you kissed, but my soul"
Judy Garland, U.S. Actress.

- Write a note for your partner telling them that you Love them, or telling them one reason why you Love them. You can do this by text, email, Facebook, Instagram, pen and paper, by sending a photo or in any other way you like.

- Organise a romantic evening picnic. Only include those foods you know your partner particularly loves, and take some outdoor, battery operated lights, or candles if you can, to decorate the setting when it becomes dark.

- Make a photo montage of the things and people you know your partner loves. You should also include yourself in it, ideally in at least one picture of the two of you together.

- Buy a small bunch of bananas, and write, "I'm bananas about you," on each one, lengthways.

- Hold hands with your partner. This becomes even more powerful if you do it whilst on a countryside walk or in a park, as it links you into a Love of Nature as well.

3. Familial Love

"You can kiss your family ... goodbye and put miles between you, but at the same time you carry them with you in your heart, your mind, your stomach, because you do not just live in a world but a world lives in you"
Frederick Buechner, U.S. Writer and Theologian.

- Give a member of your family a back scratch, (my daughter really loves these, as I've always done them for her, ever since she was a baby), a back rub, or a foot rub. Remember, Familial Love is non-sexual Love. If you do this for your partner, even if it doesn't lead to anything sexual, because of your relationship, it would be an example of Romantic Love.

- Organise a family meal and get everyone together. Of course, we often do this at special celebratory times of year such as Christmas and Easter, but do it for no reason other than just to be together. Magnify the Love by including Playful Love and playing games, whether that's board games, Pictionary, charades or any other family favourite.

- Do something, which has an emotional, financial or time cost to you, willingly for a family member. In Italy, these familial acts of Love are called, *"i sacrifici"*, (sacrifices).

- Make a photo montage of your family. You can include individual pictures of family members, or lots of group pictures. You will find that as time passes, these photos will trigger memories and become more significant and meaningful. This is especially true when loved family members move abroad or pass over and are no longer available to physically spend time with.

- Cooking your family a meal with Love, doing their washing, their ironing, the washing up, the housework and cleaning, helping with homework or any task that they need support with, when done with Love, are all acts of Familial Love.

4. Friendship Love

> *"One day Love and Friendship met for the first time.*
> *'Why do you exist when I already exist?' asked Love.*
> *Friendship smiled and replied,*
> *'To put back a smile where you've left tears"*
> Unknown Author

- One of the most common ways we show a friend that we love them is to give them a gift. Adding a note or a label, saying 'with Love', is a wonderful written reinforcement of our feelings for them.

- When a friend asks for your help, give it. Willingly and without question.

- Send a text or an email or write a card telling your friend how much you value their friendship and how much they mean to you.

- Invite your friend round for supper, take them out for lunch or find another way to treat them which is meaningful to them and which they will appreciate.

- Phoning a friend, listening to them when there's something they want to talk through, or just spending time with them and loving their company are all acts of Friendship Love.

5. Playful Love

> *"Men do not quit playing because they grow old,*
> *They grow old because they quit playing"*
> Oliver Wendell Holmes (senior), U.S. Poet.

- If you like dancing, go out dancing to a club with some friends or your partner, and really enjoy yourself. Or, put some music on at home and dance like no-one's looking!

- Spend an hour or an afternoon on your favourite hobby.

- Borrow a dog if you don't have one and take it for a walk. Find a park or a field and throw it a ball or a stick.

- Read some jokes or limericks and make some up yourself. Borrow some children's toys and play with them.

- Paint a picture, do a drawing, create a mood board or put together a photo montage of your friends and family.

6. Healthy Self-Love

> *"I love myself I do.*
> *Not everything, but I love the good as well as the bad.*
> *I love my crazy lifestyle, and I love my hard discipline. ...*
> *I love that I have learned to trust people with my heart,*
> *... I am proud of everything that I am and will become"*
> Johnny Weir, U.S. Figure Skater.

- Write a letter, (you don't have to send it), to one of your parents or best friends, telling them some of the reasons why you Love them and how they have shaped you into becoming the person that you are today.

- Start a Gratitude Diary and write a daily entry into it of at least three things you are grateful for that day.

- Write a list of all of those things that you like about yourself and that you're good at. If you can't think of any, ask your friends, family and colleagues to tell you one thing each that they think you're good at or that they value about you.

- Look at yourself in a mirror and read out loud to yourself the list that you've just written above. If you can't do it straight away with your head held high, it's ok to look down at the piece of paper and read the list. Repeat this twice a week until you can look yourself in the eye and read it.

- Write a letter to your younger self, telling them some of the things that it would be useful for them to know and giving them some useful advice which you know will help them as they grow up. The age you choose of your younger self is up to you. If you want to, you can repeat this exercise more than once for your younger self at different ages.

7. Material Love

"I am my things and my things are me ….
The accumulated external markers of who I am, … narrative prompts
for the ongoing story of my life, … and I love looking at them, love
being the person who collects this thing"
Lee Randall, US Writer and Journalist[1]

- Have a sort out at home. Find at least one thing which gives you joy when you use it or look at it and make sure that it's on display so you can see it or use it every day.

- Watch an episode of The Antiques Road Show. You will see how much love and meaning is attached to personal objects and possessions, particularly if they are heirlooms, passed down within a family through the generations.

- Find something that you love and clean it, then use it.

- Spend an afternoon wandering around antiques shops or junk shops. Find something you really love. If you can afford to, buy it. If you can't afford it, just take a photo of it. That way, it's still 'yours' in a visual way and you can retain the memory of it, and even though you never owned it you can still look at its beauty.

- Find something at home or in storage which you love, but which is damaged or broken in some way. Arrange to get it repaired, or, if you can, repair it yourself.

"My pride in what I possess IS linked to a desire for admiration and love. I hope that people visiting my home will GET me in a way that's not possible when meeting me elsewhere… my ex-husband swore that he fell for me when he saw my library and the dictionary that lives by my bed"
Lee Randall, US Writer and Journalist[1]

8. Love of Nature

*"There is pleasure in the pathless woods,
there is rapture in the lonely shore,
there is society where none intrudes,
by the deep sea, and music in its roar;
I love not Man the less, but Nature more"*
Lord Byron, Anglo-Scottish Poet.

- Buy a new plant in a pot and re-plant it lovingly in your garden or in a tub at home where it can thrive.

- Go for a 'green' walk, either in the countryside or in a park. A place where you are surrounded by green, living, things.

- The next time you see a flower, stop and look at it. Really look at it. Appreciate the delicate beauty of each perfectly crafted petal, and the curve of each flawless green leaf.

- Go for a 'blue' walk, by water. A river, a lake, the sea, a pretty stream or a reservoir. Take a notebook and pen and jot down all of the wildlife you see on your journey.

- Search the internet for photos or images of the kind of nature you love and save them to your PC. For me this is trees and woods, and also, probably because in the UK it doesn't happen very often, deep snow cover, and the crystalline beauty of a sparkling hoar frost after a freezing fog has painted everything white with its magic brush.

9. PragmaticLove

"True love doesn't happen right away; it's an ever-growing process. It develops after you've gone through many ups and downs, when you've suffered together, cried together, laughed together"
Ricardo Montalbán, Mexican Actor.

- Tidy up after a family member or your partner. The important thing is to do this exercise not begrudgingly, but rather, with genuine Love.

- Clean your car, if you have one. Not because you love your car, but because driving is safer when the windows and lights are clean and you can, 'see and be seen'.

- Do the family ironing. Again, this might be a pragmatic exercise, but doing it with Love lifts it up into something more meaningful. The same is true of the washingup!

- Take the rubbish out to the bins, or put the bins out. Replace the plastic bags If that's what you use and rinse the bins if they're dirty or smelly.

- Make a family or friendship meal with Love every step of the way. From peeling the vegetables to laying the table and serving the meal, do all things with Love.

These are only a few examples to get you started. Once you begin thinking more about Love, you will notice it much more and you will find new ways to express it and experience it all around you.

Loving Kindness Meditation
Also called *'Metta'*, meaning *'Friendship'*, Loving Kindness meditation can be described as deliberately sending positive thoughts of acceptance and well-being towards other people.

While it's not widely recognised outside direct Buddhist teachings, there are different levels of doing Loving Kindness Meditation. It can be quite difficult, I think, to go from a standing start, to firstly, Loving ourselves, to finally sending Universal thoughts of Love and well-being to those people who are hostile or who are hurting us, such as terrorist groups.

So for this reason, to make things easier for you, I've divided the guidelines for you into two parts; the first part for people you know, and the second part for those people, elements or areas that you care about but don't know personally.

Guidelines for Doing a Loving Kindness Meditation

1. Find somewhere warm and comfortable to sit down and relax.

2. Close your eyes.

3. Breathe in slowly and deeply. Hold for two seconds and then breathe out slowly. Do this 10 times. (By doing this you will already be engaging your vagus nerve).

4. Think about someone you Love. Connect with them in whichever way is the most powerful for you; visualise a picture of them, hear their voice or engage your feelings for them.

5. Think about how much you love them and accept them in every way for everything they are, and everything they have the potential to be. Wish them every joy, good health and happiness, now and at every point of time in their future.

(The length of time you choose to stay in this state is up to you, you may find that time passes quite quickly for you, and also that the engagement of your vagus nerve leads to warm feelings in your stomach or even butterflies or something similar).

6. Take these feelings and magnify them so that you are now also sending them to yourself. (I've written these guidelines this way round as many people find it easier to connect with feelings of Loving Kindness and acceptance this way, thinking about someone they Love first, rather than starting with Healthy Self-Love for themselves).

7. Now take these feelings of Loving Kindness, generosity and acceptance and apply them to other people you know. You may want to apply your thoughts to each person individually, or you may want to expand the consciousness of your thinking to various groups of people, or even to everyone you know.

…………………………………………………………………….

You might decide to stop your meditation here, with people you know. Or you might want to carry on and expand your thinking and now apply your Loving Kindness meditation more broadly. So the list below is a gently progressive one which expands until it becomes Universal.

8. Groups of people you don't know, who need help and support, such as the poor, the injured, the ill, refugees, the bereaved and the elderly. You could think of these people within one geographical location, or globally. Universal thinking is often done more easily by thinking of each point of the compass in turn; North, South, East and West, until your thinking has expanded to include the whole world.

9. Groups of people who are potentially hostile, but haven't hurt others yet, such as potential terrorists or terrorist groups who have formed but not yet acted.

10. Hostile individuals or groups who are known to have hurt others. Again, you could think of these people individually, geographically and globally.

Because Loving Kindness Meditation is a process, it can take a while to reach number 10, and not everyone will want to go that far. As a *'heart meditation'* you may find that over time, your thoughts evolve so that sending Love to those people and groups in number 10 becomes the natural and most Loving thing to do.

Chapter 6

When Good Love Goes Bad

"There is a sacredness in tears.
They are not the mark of weakness, but of power.
They speak more eloquently than ten thousand tongues.
They are the messengers of overwhelming grief,
of deep contrition, and of unspeakable love"
Washington Irving, U.S. Writer, Historian and Diplomat.

Sometimes through no fault of our own, we lose Love. Sometimes we lose Love because elements of our thinking or behaviour become incompatible with other people. Sometimes we lose Love because elements of other people's thinking or behaviour become incompatible with what we need in our lives at a particular time. And sometimes we lose Love because people change and what was once good Loving for us goes bad.

What is *'bad Love'*? It's tempting to think that all Love is good, but sadly that's not the case. Healthy Love engages our vagus nerve, releases oxytocin, serotonin and dopamine and generally makes us feel good. We either feel good because we feel relaxed and calm, or we feel good because 'Love lifts us up' and we feel elevated, inspired and excited.

Bad Love does the opposite. It makes us feel unhappy, distressed, depressed, angry, upset or scared. The sympathetic nervous system engages our fight, flight or fright response and we are flooded with the stress hormone cortisol and often adrenaline and noradrenaline as well.

Good Love nurtures and supports us. Bad Love hurts us and doesn't give us anything that we need to live a happy or healthy life.

This chapter builds on what we already know from Chapter 2 about the reasons why losing Love and bad Love are so distressing to us. From the perspective of our physical and mental well-being, both the experience of losing good Love or encountering bad Love are destructive for us physically and emotionally. We know that bad Love, and losing Love, adversely affects our body, and so learning how to minimise its damaging effects on us is an important life skill.

Distorted Love is bad Love. It includes all kinds of emotional, physical or sexual abuse, and Love which is over-controlling. Very often it's a lack of Healthy Self-Love which traps people into an unhealthy relationship involving bad Love or distorted Love. Unhealthy, 'toxic', relationships can become what relationship specialists call, 'co-dependent', where both people have an, often unconscious, emotional investment in the continuation of the destructive behaviours between them. Co-dependency can be very difficult to end as it can quickly become familiar and, therefore, comfortable, even though the relationship dynamics are damaging.

It takes tremendous self-awareness and personal courage to recognise and end an unhealthy co-dependent relationship, especially where children have also become a part of the relationship dynamic. The physical stimulation we experience from adrenaline and cortisol can become as addictive for some people as the emotional and physical highs we can encounter from Stage 1 Romantic Love.

To truly recover from an unhealthy co-dependent relationship, someone will need to re-wire their brain neurology and retrain both their brain and their body to look for, recognise and only accept more healthy patterns of good Love in their lives.

The ability to be able to recognise good, healthy Love is the single most protective factor against bad Love. Knowing how healthy Love feels, combined with the Healthy Self-Love to truly believe that we only deserve to have good Love in our lives, creates what I call the Healthy Love Triad.

The Healthy Love Triad

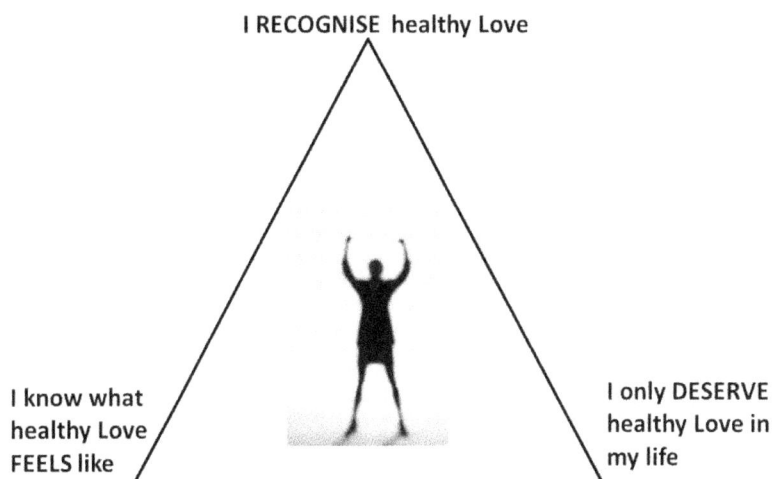

I RECOGNISE healthy Love

I know what
healthy Love
FEELS like

I only DESERVE
healthy Love in
my life

Let's move away from Distorted Love now, (abusive Love which pretends to be healthy when in reality it isn't), to consider some of the reasons why a healthy Loving relationship might change for us. People learn, grow and develop, changing over time, and a healthy Loving relationship might do one of three possible things: remain healthy and Loving, go bad but continue, or end.

Relationships end for many reasons. The most obvious reason, and the one over which we have neither influence nor control, is death.

Besides death, generally speaking, the main reason a previously healthy, Loving relationship might end, and I'm talking about all kinds of Loving relationships here, not just Romantic ones, is because one or both people are no longer getting what they need from the relationship.

I've used the word *need* very deliberately here. Wanting something within a relationship and needing something are two very different things.

Although it's not always the case, in my experience, very often wants are consciously known and can be easily identified and articulated, whereas needs can sometimes be unconsciously held. As a result, we may not be aware of what they are. It's our unconscious mind which often drives our behaviours and, as you are probably aware, it's much more powerful than our conscious mind.

Saying that you want something and yet behaving in ways that sabotage those desired goals can all be laid at the door of our unconscious mind. Weight loss, stopping smoking, taking more exercise, having the courage to be more open and honest in our relationships; all can be impaired or prevented by our unconscious.

Our unconscious mind takes full responsibility for our well-being.

One of the things that fascinates me as a coach, is that we can make our unconscious thinking, conscious. By bringing our unconscious motivations into our conscious awareness, we will invariably learn that the reasons for our self-sabotaging behaviours are all to do with keeping us physically or emotionally safe somehow, however distorted our behaviours may appear to be to our logical and rational mind.

When previously good Love goes bad, it will often be because one person's needs in the relationship are not being met in some way, either consciously or unconsciously. In addition, just to complicate things, they may not want to engage in any conversation around what's going on for them. Sometimes this is because they lack self-awareness or self-understanding, or sometimes it's because it's too uncomfortable. In which case, very often they will either put up with things as they are, or they simply walk away and start again.

Bad behaviour and bad Loving, by which I mean unhealthy, less than genuinely Loving and supportive behaviour, either directed towards someone else or turned inwards towards ourselves, can be driven by one or more of the following reasons.

What Drives 'Bad Loving' or an Acceptance of it?

- Unconscious, unmet needs.

- Unmet needs or wants we are consciously aware of.

- Not being 'brutally honest' if it would mean hurting someone.

- Having to engage in conversations we would rather avoid.

- Anger, frustration, disappointment or resentment.

- Fear. Often fear of some kind of loss.

- Clinical depression, (i.e. more than simply feeling 'low').

- A lack of respect, or worse, contempt.

- Sexual or emotional incompatibility.

- A clash of beliefs or values.

- Unhealthy Self-Love.

- Pathological narcissism or psychopathy.

- A history of previously abusive relationships, which erroneously leads someone to believe that unhealthy behaviours are either normal, or healthy.

If you remember from Chapter 2, healthy Love engages the vagus nerve and prompts the release of oxytocin and other organic, feel-good chemicals within us. All of the things listed above do the opposite of what healthy Love does to our bodies. Instead, prompting the generation and release of the stress hormone cortisol, along with adrenaline and pro-inflammatory cytokine production.

> *"Don't pity the dead Harry, pity the*
> *living, especially those who live without*
> *Love" Albus Dumbledore to Harry Potter,*
> *in*
> Harry Potter and the Deathly Hallows part II, by J. K. Rowling

"I have found the paradox, that if you love until it hurts, there can be no more hurt, only love"
Mother Teresa

Tough Love
'Tough Love' is a term used to describe a situation where unwanted behaviour is punished in some way, either by deliberate sanctions, or by the withdrawal of some kind of reward.

Within a healthy Loving relationship, rewards are freely given and are often emotional, such as the friendship itself, Love and care, respect, or someone's good opinion. Rewards can also be behavioural, such as a kind word, helping someone out, another kind of physical support, listening, or the willingness to spend time with someone. Rewards may also be financial, such as pocket money, (for children), gifts or loans, treating someone to supper, or a regular allowance for a partner or teenager for example.

Many people find Tough Love, i.e. the withdrawal of such rewards, very difficult to do. They find it very uncomfortable to behave harshly towards people they Love, even though ultimately, Tough Love is designed to support and encourage good behavior and to be for the person's own good.

It is possible however to use Tough Love *with Love*, so that we are acting from a place of Love, kindness and compassion, rather than from a place of anger, fear, pain, revenge or control. To use Tough Love *with Love*, we need to learn to sit comfortably in an uncomfortable space. It's difficult, but becomes easier with time.

Having had to use Tough Love with my own teenage daughter, I know that it's not easy. However the following suggestions might be helpful for you if you ever find yourself in a situation where you need to use Tough Love. Hopefully you will find that whatever situation or circumstances you find yourself in, will resolve themselves over time, either through the use of Tough Love, or, even better, through the use of healthy Love.

Using Tough Love *With Love*

- Be firm but fair, and above all, - be consistent.

- Be very clear what the boundaries are and exactly which behaviours are not acceptable to you.

- Also be very clear about the desired behaviours that you want.

- Make any sanctions or punishments explicit, which means being very clear about what will happen if they behave badly.

- Act immediately a boundary is broken. Don't hesitate.

- You can let them know how hurt you are, sad or disappointed, but this needs to be done in an emotionally controlled way, so that you are emotionally detached, not ranting or upset.

- Be very clear that you are not acting out of revenge, but out of Love, because ultimately, you want them to be safe.

- Be aware that they may hate you for a while, or even forever. That's an emotional cost you need to be willing to pay.

- Tell them how much you care and how much they mean to you.

- Explain gently but firmly how long the sanctions or punishments will last and when they will be lifted.

- Practise Loving Kindness Meditation. This will help you to cope and remain strong, and it will also affect the energy between you. Remember you can send Loving thoughts to a situation as well as to a person or group of people. Engage your vagus nerve to release oxytocin, so that you will genuinely feel loving towards them, even if they remain hostile, angry, upset or unrepentant.

- Keep the sanctions or punishments in place until you get the behaviours you have stated that you want.

- Reward good behaviour. Sometimes lifting the sanctions and removing the punishments will be enough, however you may want to positively reward a change in attitude or behaviour.

- Accept any apology from them with Love and good grace.

Chapter 7

How Love Can Heal You and Heal Your Life

*"The most beautiful people we have known are those who have known defeat, known suffering, known struggle, known loss, and have found their way out of the depths.
These persons have an appreciation, a sensitivity and an understanding of life which fills them with compassion, gentleness, and a deep loving concern"*
Elizabeth Kübler-Ross, Swiss Doctor and Psychiatrist.

By now you will understand how Love affects us at a cellular level. How it can influence our moods and our emotions, our thoughts and our actions. Healthy Love and good Loving are fundamentally regenerative; they can literally renew us from the inside out.

Unhealthy Love, distorted Love and bad Loving are fundamentally harmful to us; they are pro-inflammatory, emotionally as well as physically. They make us feel pain more acutely and they can delay our healing. (See Chapter 2 for the research references on this).

So how can Love heal us and heal our lives? Will any kind of Love heal us or is there some kind of magic Loving we should try first?

Random acts of kindness have been shown to make people happier. In one experiment, people were asked to perform five random acts of kindness on one specific day a week, for six weeks. Importantly, they needed to vary what they did for people rather than repeating the same thing, and the study clearly showed that those people who were deliberately kind to others felt happier than the control group of people who hadn't engaged in such random acts of kindness[1].

Laughter, playing and playfulness also have a profound effect on our brains and on our bodies. Playful Love affects us in the same ways that the other types of Love do. It energises us, relaxes us, nourishes our mind, body and soul. We should never under-estimate the power or the importance of playfulness in our lives for our emotional and physical well-being.

Interestingly, some people are naturally more serious than others and often consider playing and having fun as immature, childish and a waste of time. Yet there are other people, of all ages, who never seem to lose their sense of fun and playfulness. For them, getting older and having grandchildren is just another excuse to have fun and muck about. Their playfulness has a positive effect, not just on their physical and mental health, but also on their longevity[2]. Remember too that friendships are also are cardio-protective[3].

"One of the tasks of true friendship is to listen compassionately and creatively to the hidden silences. Often secrets are not revealed in words, they lie concealed in the silence between the words or in the depth of what is unsayable between two people"
John O'Donohue, in Anam Cara: A Book of Celtic Wisdom.

Having a better quality marriage, that's to say, more emotionally supportive, is associated with better quality health later in life[4]. Research like this suggests that, in order to be healthy and remain so, the more Healthy Love and laughter we have in our lives, the better off we will be, physically and emotionally[4-12].

We know that Love grows and expands over time. Even when our hearts are full of Love, we still have the capacity to Love more. I am sometimes asked whether we can have too much healthy Love in our lives. My answer is always that I don't think we can; with one caveat. The caveat is this; that when we Love others, we also need to remember to Love ourselves.

I've included this as a reminder that our needs and desires should not be significantly less important than the needs and wants of others. Healthy Self-Love looks like an old fashioned set of brass balance scales that sit horizontally level, with yourself on one side and others on the other.

Many people, especially women, and most particularly parents, can find this balance incredibly difficult to achieve. Our Love for others can often mean that we put ourselves at the bottom of our mental list. That isn't Healthy Self-Love; it's martyrdom!

"You yourself, as much as anybody in the entire universe, deserve your love and affection"
Buddha

Healthy Self-Love, Self-Awareness and Self-Understanding
Healthy Self-Love is the degree to which we Love and care for ourselves. As we explored in Chapter 3, there is one kind of Healthy Self-Love, but two kinds of 'unhealthy' Self-Love. Too much Self-Love can lead to feelings of entitlement, to narcissism, bullying and to aggressive, angry outbursts. Too little Self-Love can lead to a crippling lack of self-confidence, feelings of worthlessness, self-harming behaviours and other expressions of a lack of self-esteem.

There are many words that indicate Self-Love. Words such as self-respect, self-confidence, self-esteem, self-worth, self-assurance and self-regard. Self-Love also includes ideas such as being self-accepting, compassionate, and kind and forgiving towards ourselves, as these are good indicators of how much we do genuinely Love, care for and nurture ourselves.

There are three checklists which follow. They are for Self-Love, Self-Awareness and Self-Understanding. They are not designed to be comprehensive, statistically valid measures. Instead, they are designed to be quick, easy indicators of approximately how much Self-Love, Self-Awareness and Self-Understanding you currently have in your life.

The checklist for Self-Love

		No	Yes
1.	I am worth something		
2.	My happiness matters		
3.	I respect myself		
4.	I expect other people to respect me		
5.	I accept myself for who I am and what I am		
6.	I avoid people who are very critical of me		
7.	I genuinely like myself		
8.	My thoughts and feelings matter		
9.	I am my own best friend		
10.	I'm often kind to myself		

There is no 'right' score here. What I would like to suggest though, is that someone with healthy Self-Love and healthy self-regard will score somewhere between 8-10. If there are any statements that you've disagreed with, you can use them as a clue as to the areas where you may need to Love yourself more.

Without the ingredient of Healthy Self-Love, i.e. genuine feelings of care for ourselves, including self-respect and feelings of self-compassion and self-regard, no amount of self-awareness or self-understanding will make someone be kind to themselves. This is especially true if they are continually self-critical by delivering a constant stream of negative internal self-talk.

Self-Awareness is the term used to describe the conscious knowledge of our own motivations, values, thoughts, emotions, feelings, behaviours and everything else which happens within us, to us and around us. It is a pre-requisite for 'Others-Awareness', where we develop our knowledge about other people and how they are similar or different to us.

Only by developing self-awareness do we have an internal gauge by which we can measure ourselves against anyone and everyone else. It's generally thought that the development of self-awareness is an ongoing, lifelong process. It's not always a comfortable journey however, which means that not everyone is motivated to develop it.

Just because someone has self-awareness doesn't mean that they have self-understanding. Self-Understanding is subsequent to self-awareness; it happens afterwards. It's one thing to become aware of what's going on for us, particularly with regard to any patterns of thinking or behaviour that we may be running. It's quite another to fully understand the implications of those things for us. And of course, there will also be implications for the other people in our lives and we need to understand what's going on for them too.

Without Healthy Self-Love, people don't go down the route of self-awareness and self-understanding, as they're simply not motivated to learn about themselves. Blissful ignorance is often preferable to learning things which may be either uncomfortable, or may suggest that we need to change our thinking or behaviour in some way.

The checklist for Healthy Self-Awareness

		No	Yes
1.	I like learning things about myself		
2.	I can describe how I'm feeling at any moment		
3.	I recognise that not everyone thinks as I do		
4.	I can list my 5 highest values quite easily		
5.	I practise 'mindfulness' in all that I do		
6.	I'm always on a voyage of self-discovery		
7.	I'm very clear about who I am		
8.	I'm acutely aware of when I've upset someone		
9.	I'm aware of my changing energy levels daily		
10.	Being self-aware also makes me others-aware		

The checklist for Healthy Self-Understanding

		No	Yes
1.	I know why I do the things that I do		
2.	If I'm asked to explain my thinking, I can		
3.	When someone is upset with me, I know why		
4.	I can tell you what my strengths are		
5.	I understand how my moods impact on others		
6.	I always make time for self-reflection		
7.	If someone has upset me I can explain why		
8.	I understand how my weaknesses affect my life		
9.	I know what motivates me and what doesn't		
10.	I often dwell on things until I understand them		

Over the course of coaching and supporting others for more than 25 years, I have come to believe that there's a special relationship between the interaction of Self-Awareness, Self-Understanding and Self Love. It is possible to have Self-Love without the other two, and it's even possible to have Self-Awareness and Self-Understanding without Self-Love. However, those people who are really happy and successful undoubtedly have all three in their lives. More than that, they have them all in equal measure and they understand the dynamics of the interplay between them.

For example, we may have the self-awareness that we are behaving in ways that hurt ourselves and others, but we may lack the self-understanding and the self-knowledge to comprehend why it happens. Often, we don't fully know the reasons why we are driven to behave in seemingly destructive ways or how we can stop our damaging behaviours.

Even having the insight to understand that we need to change to better ways of thinking and behaving doesn't always mean that we do.

Do you remember what I said about the power of our unconscious mind in the previous chapter? Only Healthy Self-Love and having a Centred Sense-of-Self can help us, because they incorporate within them ideas of self-acceptance and forgiveness.

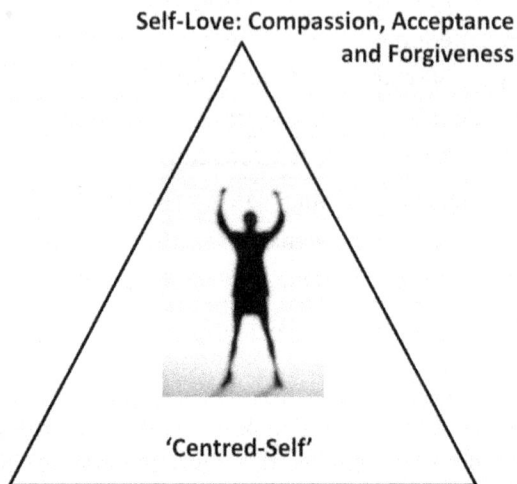

Self-Love: Compassion, Acceptance and Forgiveness

'Centred-Self'

Self-Understanding: The Implications for me are clear

Self-Awareness: I practice Mindfulness in all that I do

Having a 'Centred-Self'
Having a Centred Sense-of-Self happens when we know ourselves intimately, we understand ourselves fully, we accept ourselves completely and we can Love and forgive ourselves unreservedly.

When we are Centred, we are emotionally calm and strong. We have a robust sense of what it means to be us living our own unique life, and life's ups and downs don't throw us off balance.

This can only be achieved by the combination of Self-Awareness, Self-Understanding and Healthy Self-Love. Of all of the three elements, I have come to believe that Healthy Self-Love is the most important.

Love Heals Us: Recovery From Loss

Love can heal us in many ways. Love can heal us emotionally, by making us feel that life is worth living again, and it can heal us physically, (see Chapter 2). If you have ever experienced deep, heart-wrenching grief from loss of some kind, Love, of one type or another, is one of the very few things, if not the only thing, which will heal you.

You can throw yourself into your work, or find another distraction, but ultimately, Love is The Answer.

We all cope with loss in our own ways. For some people, familiarity with loss and grief makes new losses easier to deal with. For other people however, more loss builds on previous losses until it can become overwhelming. Bringing more Love into your life, or recognising the healthy, good Love that you already have in your life, will help to heal the dull ache of loss. Loving Reflection and Loving Kindness Meditation can both support us quite significantly through the grief process.

What follows is a message from the actor Liam Neeson, who tragically lost his wife, the actress Natasha Richardson, in a skiing accident in 2009. He posted this message was posted on his Facebook page and shared it with the world on the 2nd December 2016. I came across it as I was writing this chapter and wanted to share it with you too because it's so heartfelt.

His message was accompanied by the beautiful photo of himself and Natasha, which was taken for a magazine article some years ago, where Natasha identified and shared a picture of her favourite 'happy place'. It's a black and white photograph of Natasha in her husband's arms. He is standing behind her, with his arms protectively around her as she leans back against him. I remember reading the original article and the photograph has stayed with me in my memory ever since because it's so beautiful and evocative of a loving relationship. I couldn't reproduce it for copyright reasons, but if you look for it, once you have seen it, it will stay in your memory too.

"They say the hardest thing in the world is losing someone you love. ... Someone who showed you how to love. It's the worst thing to ever happen to anyone. My wife died unexpectedly. She brought me so much joy. She was my everything. Those 16 years of being her husband taught me how to love unconditionally. ... Life is very short. ... What I truly learned most of all is, live and love every day like it's your last. Because, one day it will be. Take chances and go live life. Tell the ones you love, that you love them every day. Don't take any moment for granted. Life is worth living".

Liam's personal quote on his Facebook page is, *"Every day I live to inspire someone. I think that's the way we should all live"*. I find his dignity and courage to be inspirational, and he has used his Love for his wife to heal himself, and to heal his life so that he can continue to live and continue to Love. This is something he continues to do every day as he carries his Love for Natasha with him in his heart.

"Your task is not to seek for love,
but merely to seek and find all the barriers within yourself
that you have built against it"
Rumi

Chapter 8

Corporate Love: Loving and Leadership

Corporate Love isn't another type of Love, after all, we have 10 of those already! Rather, the Corporate Love Model is a way of applying Love within a corporate environment.

If there was more Love for the people within organizations, (and arguably less competitiveness, greed, testosterone, selfishness and narcissism), there wouldn't be the corporate, organisational and institutional scandals, which sadly surface so regularly in the press.

Whilst some organizations are led by people who genuinely do care about the well-being of their staff, many more seem to be led and managed by those who appear to care more about balance sheets, profits, shareholder value, and personal bonuses than they do about anything else. And the irony of the whole competitive, greedy, profit-driven, back-stabbing corporate cliché, is, that in reality, by being more Loving, (that's more compassionate, kind, considerate and genuinely caring about the well-being of people), organizations could significantly increase their profits and shareholder returns[1]

Language is tricky. I designed the model and included this chapter because we need to find a new way of being able to talk about Love in the workplace, and within the corporate environment, without people confusing it with sex in the stationary cupboard!

So when I'm talking about Love at Work, let's be very clear that I'm predominantly referring to Universal Love, (or at least those parts of it which relate to kindness, compassion and a genuine concern for people's well-being). Of course, there will be Friendship Love, as having good friends at work is one of the things that makes work enjoyable, fun and meaningful. There may also be some Pragmatic Love in the mix, particularly when it comes to effective teamwork!

At the end of this chapter I'm going to share with you the results of some original research that I conducted in the Autumn of 2016 regarding the kind of leadership and management style which people say that they want in the workplace. I'm also going to share with you the kind of corporate environment that people feel they would work best in. I think the results might surprise you; they certainly weren't what I expected.

I hope that by sharing this new Corporate Love Model, you will be better able to understand why your personal style either fits well within your organisational environment or it doesn't. If by any chance your personal style doesn't fit, you will have some new insights as to the kind of supportive working environment which would suit you better, and make you a happier, more motivated, engaged and productive employee, with increased emotional fulfilment and with an enhanced sense of well-being.

Of course, what I'm saying here regarding the greater need for Love within the workplace isn't new. What is new however is the model itself, with its inherent links to our new understanding of the psychobiology of leadership, and how our underlying hormonal make-up influences our leadership and management style[2].

I'm talking here in particular about how we are driven either by testosterone or by oestrogen, and the implications that this has for our thinking, our decision-making style and our leadership and management preferences. (For more information see, *Divided by Gender, United by Chocolate: Differences in the Boardroom*[2] at *www.Unitedbychocolate.com*).

We also now have a new opportunity to talk about, *"Putting the human back into Human Resources"*, as one colleague so elegantly put it. Perhaps now is the right time to revisit what 'love' and 'loving' in all of their forms actually mean in the workplace, and to explore some acceptable ways to increase them.

Words relating to Corporate Love such as, *'kindness, compassion and genuine care,'* are being used more often now within many organizations, although sadly by no means in all. Theories of leadership and their associated models such as Ethical and Authentic Leadership, Transformational and Servant Leadership, Responsible Leadership and the new, Compassionate Leadership styles, all contain within them an inherent regard for the well-being and care of others.

The Two Axes of the Corporate Love Model
In order to begin exploring the Corporate Love Model, we need to start by considering the two axes around which it's built. On the horizontal axis is the Masculine and Feminine leadership style orientation with Conditional and Unconditional Love making up the vertical axis.

A Masculine leadership style is characterised by testosterone, which is the male hormone. Generally speaking, although there are of course exceptions, men have significantly higher levels of testosterone than women do, although everyone, both male and female, produces their own testosterone within their bodies.

Interestingly, women can also have a masculine leadership style, just as men can have a feminine leadership style. This is because the differentiating factor is in the preference for the People/Task dimension rather than with gender per se[2].

Testosterone is an amazing hormone. It's significant in the production of muscle mass and it's partly responsible for physical strength and endurance. Greater levels of testosterone are correlated with greater self-confidence and reduced levels of fear and anxiety. People with a Masculine leadership style preference are focused on goals and targets, the task at hand and results. They like to turn their attention to one thing at a time and they dislike ambiguity; they want things to be clear, straightforward and unambiguous[2]. This doesn't mean that they dislike complexity, however it does mean that they don't see the point of over-complicating things if it's not absolutely unnecessary.

The disadvantages of a Masculine leadership style also relate to testosterone, which can make some people very competitive and driven to win, focusing on the task or goal to the exclusion of everything else, including other people and their needs.

Higher baseline levels of testosterone have been shown to make people more aggressive, socially dominant, and more 'selfish', which shows not just in their behaviours at work but also in their use of language, which is less socially-oriented. In other words, people with a Masculine leadership style think more about themselves and what they want, using, *'I, me, my'* words more frequently, compared to, *'you, we, us, they, our'*, oriented language patterns[2].

Rationality, logic, process and a focus on operational numbers and financial measures with the achievement of results being paramount, are all consistent with a Masculine leadership style preference. Within leadership style theories, all of these personality traits are consistent with what's widely known as a *Transactional Style*.

In comparison, a Feminine leadership style is characterised by its nurturing, caring and supportive approach. Collaboration and the engagement and well-being of employees sits at the heart of a Feminine Leadership Style orientation. Here, arguably, people's physical and emotional well-being can be more important than the achievement of organisational goals and tasks.

Therefore the Feminine style can be considered to be a *Relational* one and it's described in leadership theories as being *Transformational* in the sense that people and organizations are transformed into something better and more meaningful by its inclusive, nurturing, supportive and engaging approach.

Whilst being predominantly collaborative and compassionate, pro-social and generous, Tough Love can also be a part of a Feminine Leadership style. However, compared with a Masculine preference, it's likely to be used considerably less often and very much as a last resort after all other avenues have been explored.

Feminine leadership is less task-focused and more creative and idealistic in its orientation, and, in contrast to the Masculine leadership style, is more 'emotional'. Biologically, it's driven by the female hormone oestrogen. Like testosterone, both men and women produce oestrogen, however, as males don't have ovaries, for them, it's produced in the bio-neurology of the brain, and, as you would expect, generally speaking, men produce significantly less of it than women generally do.

The downside of a Feminine style, at least as it's viewed from the Masculine perspective, is that sometimes the desired results and targets can take longer to achieve and results can be reduced, at least in the shorter term, (although over the longer term they can be significantly higher[1]). There is also evidence that a collaborative, less

competitive and confrontational style yields results that are more sustainable over the longer-term[1].

What we are really talking about here when we explore the influence of hormones on our leadership and management style, is the *psychobiology of Leadership*. If this is something which interests you, I have written about it in much greater depth in *Divided by Gender, United by Chocolate; Differences in the Boardroom*[2], (see *www.unitedbychocolate.com*).

The website explains the theory of *Leadership Temperament Types* and the website also gives you the opportunity to complete an online questionnaire which will identify your personal leadership style preferences if you are interested in what they might be.

In essence, from a management and leadership perspective, a people, (Feminine), versus task, (Masculine), focus can be summarised in the following diagram. As it suggests, most people will sit somewhere in the middle and, even though they may have a natural preference, will have the cognitive and behavioural flexibility to operate at both ends of the scale. Only people who have a very definite preference for one end of the continuum will struggle to work at the other end.

Moreover, generally speaking, those who are People Focused will be more flexible than those people who are Task Focused[2].

People vs Task Focus

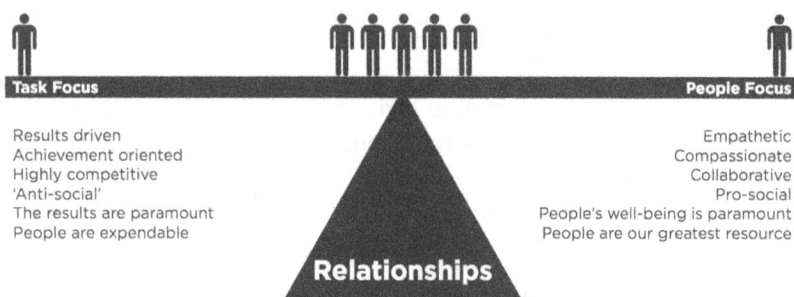

Task Focus	People Focus
Results driven	Empathetic
Achievement oriented	Compassionate
Highly competitive	Collaborative
'Anti-social'	Pro-social
The results are paramount	People's well-being is paramount
People are expendable	People are our greatest resource

Relationships

© Fiona Beddoes-Jones 2015   www.unitedbychocolate.com   www.cognitivefitness.co.uk

Now let's explore the second axis of the Corporate Love Model; Conditional versus Unconditional Regard.

Conditional Regard does what it says on the tin! The underlying assumption here is that people are neither good nor bad, but are judged wholly on their behaviours. 'Good behaviour', whatever that might mean in terms of corporate culture and organisational performance measures, is rewarded. These rewards may be financial, such as pay, a bonus and overtime, or they may be social, for example, inclusion in a project team or group of work colleagues going out after work. Or the rewards may be emotional, such as the positive attention of the manager, smiling and joking with colleagues, being thanked, or being well-regarded by line-management. Just as positive rewards can be bestowed, equally, they can be withheld or withdrawn by a leader or manager as a result of whatever the organisation considers to be poor behaviour. In addition to this, with Conditional Regard, there will be sanctions and punishments for poor performance.

This is because, as you might predict, Conditional Regard incorporates the concept of Tough Love, which we explored earlier, whereby someone will be treated harshly, even unkindly, in the belief that, in the longer term, such an approach will ultimately be better for them. Tough Love sanctions are often designed to make someone take responsibility for their own actions or to encourage them to change or modify their behaviours in some way. Not every employee responds well to Tough Love. Some may become overly stressed and be made ill by it. Tough Love can also be used by some as a legitimate reason to 'bully' some employees into more effective performance.

Unconditional Regard is an approach characterised by complete acceptance of someone's behaviour and genuine forgiveness around any mistakes or transgressions. Unconditional Regard is rare within organizations today, although it does sometimes exist, embodied within a particular leader, or within the Mission and Purpose of some charitable bodies which rely on volunteers. (See the case studies in Chapter 3 under UniversalLove).

Note: If volunteer leadership and management are of interest to you, you will find a free White Paper about it on my Cognitive Fitness website on the Resources page. The paper also includes The Volunteer Lifecycle, research on volunteer motivations and preferred job roles and a host of other useful resource references.

Unconditional Regard offers total respect for an individual and takes a holistic approach, valuing the whole person, both as they are now and as they have the potential to be in the future. It offers complete support, compassion and understanding, and is uncompromisingly generous and flexible. The major disadvantage of this approach is that individuals and organizations can sometimes manipulated or taken advantage of by less scrupulous people.

By plotting the two axes and inserting the key characteristics, the four quadrant Corporate Love Model emerges.

The Corporate Love Model

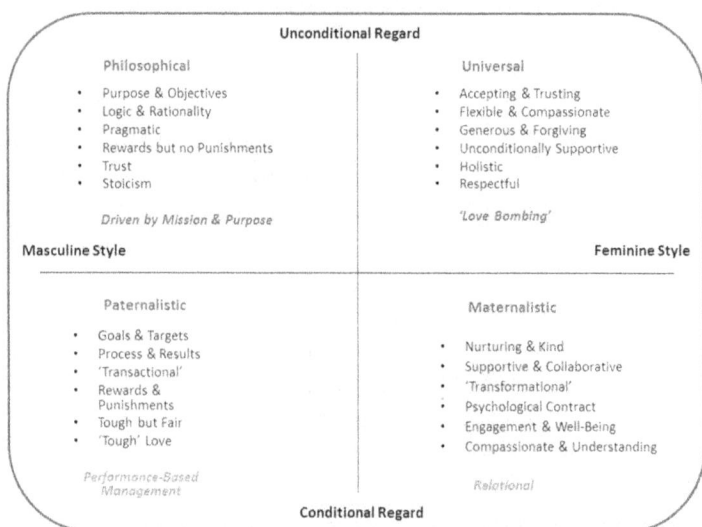

	Unconditional Regard	
Philosophical		**Universal**
• Purpose & Objectives		• Accepting & Trusting
• Logic & Rationality		• Flexible & Compassionate
• Pragmatic		• Generous & Forgiving
• Rewards but no Punishments		• Unconditionally Supportive
• Trust		• Holistic
• Stoicism		• Respectful
Driven by Mission & Purpose		*'Love Bombing'*

Masculine Style ———————————————————— **Feminine Style**

Paternalistic		**Maternalistic**
• Goals & Targets		• Nurturing & Kind
• Process & Results		• Supportive & Collaborative
• 'Transactional'		• 'Transformational'
• Rewards & Punishments		• Psychological Contract
• Tough but Fair		• Engagement & Well-Being
• 'Tough' Love		• Compassionate & Understanding
Performance-Based Management		*Relational*

Conditional Regard

If this model is too small for you to read, you will find a freely downloadable PDF version of it at *www.cognitivefitness.co.uk*

Understanding your Leadership and Management Style
Your natural preference points on the scales and your levels of flexibility to move along each of the two axes, form part of your personal underpinning philosophy of leadership.

Understanding our own personal philosophy of leadership, i.e. being self-aware around our beliefs and values regarding other people and how best to lead and manage them, is critical to becoming a good leader and manager. It links to the idea of having a Centered Sense-of-Self and is a necessary part of our own Authentic Leadership journey.

Note: if Authentic Leadership and its development are of interest to you, there's more information about it on my Cognitive Fitness website as this was the area of my PhD research.

It's NOT a Sex Thing!

I've mentioned it before, but it's so important that it's worth mentioning again; people's leadership style preference is NOT a function of their gender. Whilst it's true that gendered leadership stereotypes do hold true, i.e. most men will have a Masculine leadership Style preference and most women will have a Feminine one. However, we all know men who are particularly nurturing, caring and supportive, and we all know women who are unusually dominant, competitive, task-oriented and driven.

(If you are interested in the statistics on this, they are included in the book, which explains Leadership Temperament Types[2]).

The Potential Downsides of Each Axis

The major downside to a philosophy of Unconditional Regard is that potentially, an individual manager, or indeed an organisation, can be taken advantage of. By pursuing a course of unconditional acceptance and forgiveness, and allowing second and third, or even more chances, it's possible that bad behaviours and poor attitudes, because they go unchallenged and unpunished, may persist.

Because Conditional Regard is transactional in nature, some people will only give what's contractually expected of them and no more. (Giving more of ourselves than is actually contractually agreed is known as *Discretionary Effort*, and involves the activities and attitudes we give the organisation that we're not paid or recompensed for). In addition, some people may be hurt if Tough Love and sanctions are used against them and they feel that they don't deserve to be treated in a harsh way.

The major drawback of a Masculine Leadership Style is that with its focus on goals and targets, procedures, objectives and results, the well-being and importance of people somehow gets lost in the mix. At its worst, people can be made to feel like numbers or disposable assets who are not valued; either by their leaders and managers or by their organisation.

These thoughts and feelings, because of something called *emotional contagion*, may become common amongst the workforce who respond to this transactional approach by simply doing what they are paid to do and no more. Their discretionary effort is reduced to zero, as are their levels of engagement and motivation.

Potentially, where a Feminine leadership style is predominant, and people's well-being is paramount, sometimes goals or targets may be not be achieved and desired corporate results can be delayed over the short term. A Masculine style is predominant in business today, and in a world of quarterly reporting with the constant scrutiny of performance management, delayed results are rarely acceptable.

The Advantages of each Corporate Love Quadrant
A Paternal Style
(Masculine Leadership Style with Conditional Regard)
A Paternalistic approach is usually operational rather than strategic in its orientation. With its focus on goals, targets, process, procedures and objective measurements, a Paternalistic Style, to which the closest description is *Performance-Based Management*, will always get results.

It even gets the best out of some people. That's to say, people who are generally task-focused and who respond well to clear rules and defined boundaries. There is an emphasis on control and on reporting, so it's easy to compare current with past performance and to build on it. Systems, procedures and protocols will all be in place, so it's a transparent, tough but fair, organizational culture.

A Maternal Style
(Feminine Leadership Style with Conditional Regard)
Employees will feel well cared for, nurtured and supported within a Maternalistic culture where the focus is *Relational,* i.e. people-focused on compassion, understanding and collaborative working to achieve organisational results. Very often rewards and benefits will be flexible, or even designed so employees can put together their own unique package, which suits their personal work/life balance.

Even though sanctions will still be in place to manage poor performance, the ethos will always be on taking a supportive and nurturing approach. The *psychological contract*, (unwritten understandings about the relationship), is recognised as being critical to the employment relationship, which is viewed as being mutually beneficial and ideally, a long-term one.

A Philosophical Style
(Masculine Leadership Style with Unconditional Regard)
This is the quadrant where many charities and Charitable Trusts sit, as they are driven by the ideals of their stated Mission or Purpose. Here, they often rely on volunteers to help them achieve their objectives. The organisation takes a pragmatic and stoic approach where people are trusted to perform and there are very few, if any sanctions in place if they don't.

The organisation may have quite well-defined systems and procedures in place to manage things. However, it's very difficult to discipline volunteers as, by definition, they are not employees and have no contract of employment. Therefore, non-performance or poor behaviours are often accepted and seemingly overlooked.

A Universal Style
(Feminine Leadership Style with Unconditional Regard)
A nurturing, caring and supportive culture where people are trusted absolutely to do their best. These are the kind of organizations that are sometimes so progressive the employees decide upon their own pay and benefits. Everyone genuinely feels valued and the inclusive and collaborative working environment is one where people talk about being part of a 'family'. Employees often feel passionately about the organisation and feel immensely proud of what it has achieved[1].

Morale and motivation tend to be high, as are engagement and discretionary effort. Turnover is low as is employee absenteeism. Measures of well-being and happiness are also high. Mistakes, while not encouraged, are forgiven and seen as learning opportunities.

Employees feel accepted and genuinely valued for all that they are and they are encouraged to bring, 'all of themselves' to work; that's to say their life skills, hobbies and interests, and those things which make them unique and special as human beings. Employee diversity is genuinely lived in the organisation, it's not simply a paragraph laminated in the Values Statement.

The 2016 Research on 'Love in the Workplace'
I expect that as you've been reading this chapter you will have been thinking about your own personal preferences and where you think you might sit in the model. So now let me share with you the results of the research I did in the UK in the autumn of 2016. When I put the research out on the internet to ask for participants, I badged it as a study about Leadership Style preference. I didn't mention Love at all because I didn't want to adversely influence people's expectations, their responses or their willingness to take part.

Over 300 people contributed to the study, 96% of whom have, or have had, a management or leadership role. There was a very slight gender bias towards women; 56% compared with 44% of men taking part, and 88% worked within the UK rather than any other country in Europe. 92% were of working age, between 26-65 years old.

I received 126 responses within the first 24 hours of starting the study. One of the fascinating things for me was that after only 26 responses a pattern began to emerge. This pattern remained completely consistent throughout the whole study. When patterns emerge and remain stable, we can be pretty sure that we've found something real, and that adding more people to the project won't change the results. So I closed the study after we had passed the 300 people mark, which is double the size of population sample we generally need for statistically valid results.

Only after talking about Leadership Style for a while within the research questions did I introduce the idea of 'Love' in the workplace. I very clearly defined 'Love' as, *"Compassion, caring and a genuine regard for people's well-being."* Which of course you will recognize as being a part of Universal Love from Chapter 3.

Results of the 2016 Research

1. Overwhelmingly, **96%** of people agreed that they would work harder for an organisation which they felt genuinely cared about them and their well-being. This gives a very clear message that people want Universal 'Love' at work, and want to *be* 'Loved' at work; they perceive it to be something which is not just acceptable, but desirable.

2. The majority of people were dissatisfied with the level of warmth and care displayed where they worked. **70%** felt that their well-being at work would be improved if there were more 'Love' within the culture of their organisation. There is some good news however, with **30%** of people feeling that there is already enough genuine caring and support within their working environment.

3. Regarding working culture, **70%** of people said that they would prefer a *'collaborative & supportive'* working environment, which is a Feminine leadership style, driven by oestrogen. Only **26%** of people said that they would prefer to work within an organisational culture which was *'task-focused and goal-oriented'*, which we know to be a Masculine leadership style, driven by testosterone.

4. Interestingly, people wanted the opposite from their direct line manager. **70%** of people said that they would prefer a manager with a Masculine leadership style, i.e. *'tough but fair'* and *'logical and pragmatic'*. Only **26%** of people said that they would prefer a manager with a Feminine leadership style, i.e. *'nurturing and kind'* and *'unconditionally supportive'*.

Therefore there's a very clear dichotomy here between the supportive 'feminine' cultural environment people say they want to work in, compared with how they want to be led and managed directly, which is in a logical and pragmatic, task-focused and goal-oriented, 'masculine' way.

5. 65% of people felt that there's sometimes a lack of Love within the culture of their own organizations. This may go some way towards explaining why 83% believe that leaders and managers should be formally taught how to 'Love' their staff. That is, to be considerate, to genuinely care for their wellbeing, and to be compassionate and supportive.

6. Regarding Tough Love, **87%** of people said that they would prefer not to have to use Tough Love at work if they could avoid it and still get the same results. Moreover, **50%** of people, (remembering that **96%** of them have, or have had, a management or leadership role), said that they find Tough Love difficult to implement at work. Only **41%** reported that they are comfortable with using Tough Love at work.

The Courage to Lead
Now a word about Courage, because it seems to me that we all sometimes need courage at work to stand up for what we believe in. This is particularly the case if we are naturally compassionate, Loving and nurturing, and we're working in a Masculine culture of performance management.

Courage …. from old French *cuer* meaning *heart*

1. The quality of mind and spirit that enables a person to face danger with bravery.

2. (*Obsolete*) The heart as the source of emotion. Compassion, empathy

3. Acting in accordance with one's beliefs and values in the face of criticism or danger.

While it might be obsolete now in our everyday language, having *courage* used to be associated with having *heart*; from a Universal, compassionate and empathetic perspective.

One of the things I learned about myself in the course of completing my PhD in authenticity and Authentic Leadership, is that Courage is one of my highest values. I always notice people who are physically or emotionally brave and yet who are also kind, considerate and compassionate. I've reflected on it quite a lot over the years, and I've come round to thinking that perhaps it's because they are quite rare and almost uniquely flexible. After all, they are the modern, living embodiment of both the masculine, testosterone-driven Warrior and Protector, and yet also of the feminine, nurturing Carer.

"Courage is the ladder on which all the other virtues mount"
Clare Boothe Luce, U.S. Congressman and playwright 1903-1987

Implications of the 2016 'Love in the Workplace' Research.

1. It seems that there's an enormous potential gap in employee engagement and productivity, which could be tapped into by a more 'loving' and compassionate leadership style.

2. We need more Love in the workplace; more genuine caring, more kindness, more consideration, more compassion and more unconditional regard. It's what people want.

3. The cultural leadership style environment which employees want from their organisation, compared with what they want from their direct line manager may be very different.

4. It's quite rare for leaders and managers to have an equal preference for both a masculine and a feminine leadership style. Most people have one clear preference and need to work on developing their flexibility to use the other one.

5. There appears to be both a need, and a desire, for leadership and management development programmes to include 'Love' and 'Tough Love' within them, which is not currently being addressed within organizations.

"People don't care how much you know,
Until they know how much you care"
Theodore Roosevelt, 26th President of the USA.

As a result of these implications, a number of suggestions emerge:

Suggestions to Organisations and Human Resources, (HR), Directors

1. Think very carefully about the Corporate Love Model and the kind of organisational culture you have, compared to the kind of organisational culture you want or need. What you have will often be driven by the Leadership Style preferences of the CEO and the Board, and may not be the most appropriate one!

2. Consider reviewing your Employee Engagement Survey responses from the perspective of 'Love'. What is the feedback and the messages your people are giving you?

   By being more 'Loving' and engaging your staff you will be able to significantly increase your engagement figures and people's well-being, make productivity improvements, reduce absenteeism and turnover, become more creative and collaborative and reduce expenditure costs in many areas[1].

3. Don't do things *to* your workforce; involve them and engage them in the process. Be honest and authentic regarding your motivations and communicate with them effectively every step of the way. Your absence and turnover figures will be an indicator as to how well you are doing.

4. Consider including Leadership Temperament Types[2] in your management and leadership development programmes. When people have a copy of their own profile, it gives them a frame of reference and a common language to work more effectively with their colleagues, and enables them to develop themselves.

5. Find the right language. You need to develop a comfortable way of being able to talk about caring deeply, of 'Love' and 'Loving', of compassionate regard and of consideration for people's well-being in the organisation. Being 'Loved' and genuinely cared about really matters topeople.

6. Teach people how to 'Love' each other and how to 'Love' their staff in ways that feel comfortable and appropriate for them and the organizational culture.

   You will particularly need to include things on boundaries and Tough Love, as many people, (**59%** in my research), find Tough Love difficult to use effectively at work. These things are life skills. They are also relationship skills which will make a dramatic difference to your employees' lives in all kinds of ways. Re-read Chapter 2 if you don't believe me!

And Finally, The Million Dollar Question …

This is the question which I am asked every time I talk about the Corporate Love Model. "How?" Is the question. More specifically,

"How can we have both a Masculine and a Feminine leadership style so that we can give our employees what they want, when the two styles appear to be soopposite?"

I'm going to resist saying that Love is The Answer here, although in a way, of course it is!

Using the metaphor of a family, we are very adept at incorporating both masculine and feminine styles within a family group, even if it's the mother who thinks in a classically masculine, task-oriented way and the father who is the more gentle and nurturing. What I'm saying here is that firstly, we already intuitively know the answer to the question and how to make it work effectively, and secondly, it's the thinking which is important here and not physical gender[2].

The ONLY starting point for organisations is to actually GENUINELY care for their employees enough in the first place to want to support them, (more 'tone from the top' here). Then they have to provide the organisational infrastructure as a framework to make performance possible through the appropriate processes and procedures which need to be supportive and flexible.

Finally, they have to create a culture of, 'Loving Kindness', so that values such as genuinely caring are encouraged and rewarded, (emotionally rather than financially). If this is something that you want to create for your organiation, simplifying your thinking around the People/Task continuum will ensure that you don't focus on one side at the expense of the other. You need to embrace both equally and build both of them into the culture of the organisation.

A word of warning here; we know that corporate culture is driven by the leadership style of the people at the top. We also know that generally speaking, stereotypically, the people at the top will be there because they are highly competitive, performance focused, driven, numerate and results-oriented[2]. In other words, they are very Masculine in their leadership style, (regardless of whether in gender terms, they are male or female).

Very often, these people are at the extreme end of the Task continuum with very little cognitive or behavioural flexibility and very little Emotional Intelligence. Because they don't understand it, they tend to perceive caring as, *"soft, wishy-washy and pointless"* which doesn't contribute to bottom-line profits. How wrong they are![1]

So you mustn't allow these people to ride roughshod over the culture of the organisation if you want the organisation to continue to exist, and to thrive after they have moved on, (bearing in mind that the average tenure of a CEO seems to be in the region of two short years!).

They move on, I believe, because their style doesn't work in terms of building harmony, collaboration, engagement, creativity or, ultimately, in terms of building any kind of sustained performance.

In summary, the answer to the question is to create a caring, nurturing, understanding, generous and supportive corporate culture, (from the Feminine 'soft' style), which is underpinned by the appropriate systems, procedures, processes and organisational infrastructure, (from the Masculine, 'hard' style), to enable your managers and leaders to be kind, and also, importantly, to be fair.

When kindness, collaboration, generosity and support become organisational values, people will be delighted to be able to use them. In other words, you are creating an environment that takes the very best from a Masculine style, and the very best from a Feminine style, regardless of the physical gender of your managers and leaders and their personal Thinking Styles[3]. When high performance expectations are also built into the mix, the organization and the people in it will thrive and flourish.

If, as a leader or manager, you are mindful of the effect and impact that your attitude, thinking and behaviours have on those around you, and if you do your best to do all things with Love, then you won't go far wrong.

Note: Please remember that there is more freely downloadable information and a larger PDF version of the Corporate Love Model on the Cognitive Fitness website at *www.cognitivefitness.co.uk*

Chapter 9

In What Ways is Love the Answer? Case Studies

"Not everything has to change for everything to change"

This chapter uses amalgamated case studies of real people's stories to give you insights into the ways in which understanding and using the 10 different kinds of Love can help us within our relationships. The format of the Case Studies is to briefly summarise the issue and then to explore the ways in which understanding and applying some of the different kinds of Love could help the situation and make a real difference to the lives of the people in the scenario.

The thoughts and suggestions offered here are given purely from my perspective. If the situation was told to you by a friend or a colleague, your thoughts and suggestions may well be different to the thoughts which I have, and to the suggestions and advice which I offer. As you read through each case study example I would invite you to consider the question, *"In what ways is Love the answer here?"* Having read the rest of the book you might be surprised at the thoughts and insights which occur to you.

Case Study 1
My mother is dying and I wish I could care but I don't feel anything. I'm so ashamed of myself.

My mother has always been very critical of me. Even as a child I don't ever remember her hugging me, kissing me or telling me that she loved me. My father once bought me a kitten for my birthday but she gave it away saying that it was dirty and had fleas. I was really happy when I managed to escape to University, but I struggled to fit in and I often felt lonely and isolated. It was made worse because I really missed my dad, but my mother seemed delighted that I was away from home so she could have my father's attention all to herself again.

I never married because I found it difficult to form relationships and I was scared of having children and not loving them. I didn't want to do to them what my mother had done to me. So I focused on my career instead. After my father died I moved away although I tried really hard to be a dutiful daughter. I visited regularly even though I hated every minute of the time I spent there. Now my mother has dementia and is dying of cancer but I'm ashamed to say that I just don't care. I don't seem to feel anything but relief that she will soon pass away and be gone; out of my life forever. I'm hoping that then I will be able to rebuild my life somehow. I feel like an awful person and the worst daughter in the world.

I'm so sorry that your mother's love for you was a jealous one and that it's affected your life so monumentally; it's coloured everything that you've done since you were a teenager. The relationship you have described from your mother is an emotionally cold one, the kind some relationship counsellors would call emotionally abusive, and it's prevented you from forming loving adult relationships, at least up until now. In your letter you describe your shame, but reading between your words, I can detect that there's also an undercurrent of anger, albeit that you've buried it so deeply that you appear to have hidden it even from yourself.

There is no need to feel ashamed, or to feel like an awful person. You are not an awful person and your suppressed anger is completely understandable. We often feel angry as a result of being hurt, and your mother's behavior towards you over the years must have been very hurtful. So now you say that you have shut off all of your emotions towards your mother and don't feel anything but relief that she will soon be gone from your life. Shutting off your feelings for your mother will of course stop you from feeling any anger towards her, but it will also stop you from feeling any love for her, or even normal human compassion for the sick and elderly.

After she has passed away you may find that once you feel 'safe' again you will reconnect with your emotions and you may deeply regret anything between you which was left unsaid. You may also find yourself grieving for the kind of loving and caring relationship that you never had with your mother, and now never will have.

Cutting off your emotions, whilst it's a completely understandable self-protection mechanism, is ultimately self-defeating as it prevents you from feeling positive emotions as well as the negative ones you are avoiding. It may help in the short-term, but it's unlikely to help you in the longer-term. If you really want to heal yourself, and have healthy, successful loving relationships in the future, you need to learn to love yourself. Learning to love ourselves is a journey of many steps, so take one step at a time and remember how much your father loved you. This will give you the springboard that you need. Good luck in your journey.

Case Study 2
My husband has been having an affair.

I've just found out that everything I thought was sacred in my marriage has been a sham. I feel such a fool for believing my husband's stories of pressure at work, having to work late and mid-week conferences. I found the evidence on a secret phone including pictures of my husband and his mistress together … I recognise his private body parts. I can't eat, I can't sleep, I can't work; I just feel sick. I'm like a zombie who sobs all day. Only having to look after our two young children gives me any meaning in my life and makes it possible to get up in the morning. I haven't confronted my husband yet and he doesn't seem to suspect that anything is wrong. What do I do? I love my husband but I hate him at the same time. There's nothing left to save of my marriage, it's over, but I don't know what to do next.

Finding out that you have been betrayed by your husband in so graphic a way must be incredibly painful. Loss of any kind is one of the most difficult things which we ever have to deal with, and your letter and your tears suggest that you are both in shock and also grieving for the devastating loss of your marriage. That you say you hate your husband is completely understandable, yet you also say that you still love him.

It is possible to love and hate someone at the same time, especially when the love came first. Hold on to the love, because where there is love there is hope.

Some marriages do survive the discovery of an affair, especially when children are involved and both parents have a commitment to them. It's too early to say whether your marriage will be one of them, but it may be. At some point you are going to have to decide whether to confront your husband and tell him that you know about the affair, or ignore it in the hope that it will burn itself out and end naturally. Of course, even if it does, there's no guarantee that your husband won't simply go on to find another mistress.

You might not like what I'm going to say, but I do just wonder what it is that your husband gets from his lover that he's not getting at home? Is it possible that with all the responsibilities and effort required from parenting two young children that the pair of you no longer have the time for each other that you used to have? Time for conversation and listening to each other, time to play and have fun together, time for the emotional and sexual intimacy which is the hallmark and bedrock of a healthy marriage? Whilst it doesn't make his behavior acceptable, perhaps there might be a way of at least understanding why he has behaved in the ways that he has.

You still love your husband, and I'm sure that he loves you. You are, after all, not just his wife but the mother of his children, whom you both love. There is a bond between you which is stronger than the legal contract of your marriage and that's worth cherishing.

There are many ways to have a happy marriage. And one of the things that they all have in common is that there is open, honest and loving communication between people within an environment of trust. If you do decide to confront your husband or even to end your marriage, the one thing that you are both going to need to do is to talk to each other. You have been very hurt and whilst this is currently causing you to cry, there may come a time when it also makes you become very angry. Anger is understandable in your situation, and it gives us energy, but it also causes us to lash out and hurt others so please be careful what you say and when you say it. I'm mentioning this because the danger is that the people who are hurt the most will be your children, something which I'm sure neither you, nor your husband, would want.

If you and your husband want to find out what killed your marriage, you are going to need to work together to solve its murder. You will need to take your marriage apart piece by piece, like the jigsaw puzzle of a crime scene, so you can look at each piece individually and examine it to see how it contributes to the whole picture of your marriage. Only then will you be able to see where the missing pieces are, and only then will you be able to rebuild it, together, piece by piece. You have the opportunity to rebuild your marriage so that it's better and stronger than it evidently was before.

I will leave you with a quote which I use within couples counselling and mediation. It suggests putting your pain, anger, hurt and ego to one side, so you can deal calmly with the situation and resolve it. It's not easy, in fact it's very difficult, but I can promise you, it is worth it. I really hope that you can work this out between you and save your marriage. If you can do this with love, compassion, understanding and forgiveness, then you won't go far wrong.

"Out beyond ideas of wrong doing and right doing there is a field.
I'll meet you there."
Rumi

Case Study 3
My fiancée stays in bed all day and I don't know what to do.

My boyfriend and I met at university and dated for 3 years before getting engaged and moving in with each other. He used to be so positive and full of life, but now, unless he has to go to work, he just stays in bed all day or plays on his x-box. I work too, but now I have to do all the cooking and the cleaning or it doesn't get done. We used to go out a couple of times a week but he always says that he's too tired. Our sex-life has dwindled to nothing and I'm seriously wondering whether to stay in the relationship. I want to support him, but he says that he doesn't want to talk about it and that I should stop nagging. The tenancy agreement on our flat is up for review soon, should I tell him that it's over between us or should I keep trying to make it work? If we were married I wouldn't leave him so perhaps I shouldn't be thinking about it now?

Are you sure that if you were married that you wouldn't leave him? What would you do differently if you were married? It sounds like you've been supportive of him, but unfortunately your supportive behaviour hasn't changed either his attitude or his actions, so maybe you need to try something else. I think you intuitively know this, which is why you're suggesting ending the relationship. This is a form of Tough Love; where we use sanctions or punishments, (or threats of using them), to try to get people to change.

Sometimes Tough Love works and sometimes it doesn't. Feeling that you're forced to use it doesn't mean that you don't love your fiancée, or that you love him any less, just that you think you've tried everything else and that Tough Love is the only thing that you have left to do. In this instance, Tough Love effectively means saying, *"I'm done. I've tried everything else, I'm walking away, I might love you, but as long as you keep doing what you're doing, you're on your own"*.

But I'm going to challenge your thinking a little bit. Have you really tried everything else? The description of your fiancée's behaviours suggest that he may be suffering from depression. He will need to see his GP either to rule it out, or to discuss his treatment options. Treatment is usually medication, conversations with a therapist, or a combination of the two. Can I suggest that you encourage your fiancée to see his GP and a counsellor, and only if he refuses do you go down the Tough Love route. I hope that it all works out for you.

Case Study 4
I love my girlfriend and want to propose, but my parents don't like her .... should we get married?

Usually I ask my parents for advice but I can't in this instance as my question involves them. I met my girlfriend at university five years ago and we've been together now for three years. I love her very much, to me she's perfect. We started living together six months ago and I want to propose to her but my parents don't like her. They don't seem to think that she's good enough for me, but I do and surely it's my choice to make not theirs. I've always been close to my family and it's tearing me apart to think that I might have to choose between them or her. What should I do?

Your love for both your girlfriend and your family is clear from your letter, as is the anguish that you are currently experiencing. You're obviously very close to your family and I'm curious as to why they think that your girlfriend isn't good enough for you, as it's clearly not the way which you feel about her. Whilst she's been in your life for five years, your parents haven't known her for as long as you have, and of course, as young adults, you will both have grown and matured a lot over the past few years.

You say that your girlfriend is 'perfect'. This suggests that you are still in the 'honeymoon' period of your romantic relationship. It also suggests that you see an idealized version of her, rather than the reality of how she actually is. In reality no-one is perfect; we all have our strengths and weaknesses as we're only human, and that means to occasionally make mistakes and be flawed.

You haven't mentioned when you first introduced your girlfriend to your parents, but perhaps they are allowing their initial impressions of her to colour their current opinions? No one likes being judged and found wanting, so perhaps your girlfriend has unconsciously picked up on their feelings towards her which may mean that she avoids them or isn't as loving towards them as you know her to be?

It might seem like a strange thing for me to say, but becoming engaged and actually getting married are two, very different, things. Whilst becoming engaged is an intention to marry, it's not a legally binding contract in the same way that a marriage is. Ending an engagement if it doesn't work out, whilst still very painful, doesn't involve lawyers, possible legal wrangling over joint possessions and finances, or court orders for shared custody of children or animals. I know I'm painting a bit of a bleak picture here, but sometimes it's useful just to take a reality check and do some 'worst case scenario planning' to examine our thoughts and feelings. If you were ever to divorce, would your girlfriend fight you for all that she's legally entitled to, or would she be kind and loving and do her best to continue to be supportive as you both try to navigate the very difficult waters of divorce?

Marriage joins two families, not just two people. If you do decide to become engaged, how your girlfriend interacts with your family to plan the wedding will also give you big clues as to whether she's the right woman not just for you, but for your family as well. Your thoughts around these questions will help you to clarify whether becoming engaged and subsequently married are the right steps forward for you and your girlfriend. Either way, I wish you well.

Case Study 5
My Father-in-Law makes our lives a misery and I hate him for it.

My Father-in-Law is a horrible man. He bullied his wife since they married 46 years ago and he was very strict with my husband while he was growing up. He ignores our two children who are his only grandchildren and I hate him for upsetting them. My husband is scared of him and won't stand up to him about his selfish behaviour. His wife seems to love our children, but is too scared to talk to me about anything other than the weather which makes me disappointed in her as well as in herson. I seem to be becoming angry all the time with everyone apart from our children. This isn't what I signed up for and not the kind of marriage I want.

I'm losing respect for my husband over it and I'm worried that it's going to affect my own marriage. What can I do to save my marriage and my relationship with my in-laws?

It's an awful thing to see pain and hurt on our own children's faces, and not surprisingly, as a mother and a wife, you want to wave a magic wand and fix everything that you feel is wrong within your family and your extended family. It's very sad to think that the bullying and insensitive behavior of one man has been able to adversely affect the lives of so many people, including your life. The reasons for your father-in-law's cold and bullying behavior aren't important, although perhaps by understanding them better you might find yourself feeling more compassionate towards him rather than just the anger and hate you currently feel.

There are a number of ways you could approach the issues you've identified but I'm going to be bold and suggest that there is one approach which stands head and shoulders above the rest of them. Please take a moment to think about the following questions: What would be the most loving and kind things to do here? How can you be your best self in this situation and show others in what it means to be loving? In other words, in what ways is Love the answer here?

Your husband needs your Love and support. Becoming angry at him simply doesn't help, in fact, it's worse that that; it's very destructive as you're effectively punishing him for being himself, which simply hurts him more. Surely he experienced enough of that in his childhood from his father? He needs your strength and your love to make him strong so that you can stand united. Being married is to be a part of a very special team which works together; a team which your children are also a part of. I'm going to make some very specific suggestions here regarding how you can bring more Love and compassion to your current circumstances. I'm sure that you can adapt them if you feel that you need to.

- Sit down with your husband at a time when you won't be interrupted and tell him how much you love him and that you're a team and that he has your complete support. Say that you understand how difficult he must find it to stand up to his father and how proud you are of him that he doesn't behave in the same ways to your own children. Remind him of the reasons why you fell in love with him and give him at least three examples of what a wonderful husband and father he is. (There may be some tears during this conversation, possibly from both of you. However, they are healing tears, so let them flow if they do come, you will both feel better for expressing and sharing them).

- Sit down with your children and say that you want to explain some things about their grandfather. Tell them that you're sure he loves them very much but that because of his own upbringing he finds it difficult to express his feelings for them. Also tell them that as men get older, changes in their brain mean that they can become rather grumpy and bad-tempered, and that they can't help it. (Fascinatingly, this is known as *Grumpy Old Men Theory* and you will actually find it on the internet if you look for it!).

- Create some opportunities for you and your extended family to all be together, such as a Sunday Lunch for example. Don't expect active participation from your father-in-law, but rather, be loving and have fun around him. Allow him to be an observer and hopefully at some time he will decide to become involved. If he's grumpy, take a step back and give him some space but continue to have fun and be loving. I'm sure that he will eventually become more pleasant to be around.

- Start doing Loving Kindness Meditation. Start your thinking with your children as you I'm sure you Love them unconditionally. Then extend your thinking to your husband, your friends, other members of your family whom you do like, and then finally to your Father-in-Law. I'm sure you will find that your attitude towards him softens and your anger towards him dissipates a little.

Paradoxically, your Father-in-Law has given you an opportunity to strengthen your marriage and your relationship with your husband. Be your best self and let others follow your lead.

Case Study 6
My son thinks that I love his sisters more.

This is one of the hardest things I've ever had to admit, but I've never been a very hands-on father. My parents loved me I'm sure but they weren't very demonstrative and I find it difficult to express my feelings. I love my children and I've always tried to treat them equally, but there's no doubt that I find it easier to spend cuddle-time with my younger daughters than I do with my son. I love them all the same amount but my son has accused me of loving his sisters more. I denied it because it's not true but I don't know what else to say to him. Please help me repair my relationship with my son.

Putting your story and your feelings in a letter to me has been understandably difficult. Writing things down however is always useful as it helps us to clarify our thoughts and the emotions which surround them. From what you've said, I'm unsure whether you find it difficult to cuddle your son because he is older than your daughters, or because he is a boy. In a way, this is less relevant than the fact that he has noticed and challenged you on it; and it's clearly something which you both obviously find distressing.

You say that your son has rejected your verbal assurances that you love all of your children equally. Perhaps he feels that your words don't match your actions, as you yourself readily admit that you physically cuddle your daughters more. Perhaps actions would speak louder than words here? Does your son want you to cuddle him more? Or perhaps he would like to spend some more quality, alone time with you, just the two of you?

I can assure you that all is not lost and that you will be able to repair the relationship with your son. That's what families do; they may fall out, but then they, (usually), forgive and reset the relationship.

There is a new parenting technique you may not have heard of which I'm sure will help you both. It's called Love Bombing, and is a simple and effective technique for repairing and resetting the parent-child bond which involves spending time with your child in a way where they have 100% of your emotional and physical attention. The intention is to make your child feel completely loved and secure in your love for them and in the relationship that you have with them.

I would recommend that you read *Love Bombing: Resetting Your Child's Emotional Thermostat,* by the psychologist Dr. Oliver James. I wish you both all the very best.

Case Study 7
I've developed feelings for my best friend and now I'm confused.

Me and my best friend have been inseparable since we were at junior school. We do everything together; we see each other every day at college and spend most evenings and weekends together too. We often date boys in a foursome and we talk about boys all the time. But recently I've begun looking at her differently and I've noticed how beautiful she is. Now I'm really confused. I'm sure I'm straight but I know that I love her more than anyone else. I'm so confused and I can't talk to her about it. It's causing a rift between us. She keeps asking me what's wrong but I just can't tell her. Am I gay after all? I just don't know what to do.

Growing up from being a child into a young adult can often be a confusing time. There are many things to experience and to learn. Understanding our own sexuality is a part of our personal journey into adulthood. For many people, our sexual preferences are apparent to us from a young age. For others of us our sexual preferences are more fluid and may even change as we mature into ourselves. Your letter suggests that you consider yourself to be heterosexual, although you also find your best (girl) friend to be beautiful. Interestingly, what you haven't said is that you find your girlfriend to be sexually attractive.

There are different kinds of Love. I'm sure that you love your parents for example and your brothers and sisters if you have them. The love you feel for the members of your family is called Familial Love, and you love them without feeling sexual attraction for them. It sounds to me as if you love your girlfriend in a similar way, although because she's not family, your relationship would fall under the category of Friendship Love. All love involves strong emotions and both Familial and Friendship Love can be very powerful.

It's completely natural that we would find the things and the people we love to be beautiful. And it's also completely natural that you would feel love for your best friend. It seems to me that you *Love* her, but you're not *in Love* with her. That's the subtle difference between Friendship Love and Romantic Love. Perhaps you could have a conversation with your girlfriend about the different kinds of Love you each have in your lives and how much your friendship means to you both. I feel sure you will find that your friend loves you too from a loving Friendship perspective and that your current confusion will be resolved.

Case Study 8
My partner died three years ago – will I ever learn to Love again?

Since my partner and soul mate died unexpectedly approximately three years ago life's been very difficult. For the first few weeks I was sort of ok, what with arranging the funeral and speaking to people. Then I kind of focused on sorting out the money stuff and her clothes and I kept busy. The only way to get through the days was to pretend that she was just on holiday and would be back soon. Whenever I thought about the finality of death and of never seeing her again I just cried and cried and couldn't get out of bed. I lost 60 kilos because I couldn't eat, I couldn't sleep, couldn't think straight at work, ... I was a mess.

Slowly, slowly, I got used to a new normal, ... life without her. But everything seems so meaningless now. I used to have a future, ... we used to have a future, ... but now when I try and look into the future, there's nothing there; just a big hole where she used to be. Work's been a life-saver to be honest, and I even laughed for the first time in years the other day. But then I started sobbing again because I thought of her and how much she would have enjoyed the joke too, ... but of course she can't and she never will.

I'd never understood the term 'mad with grief' before, but now I do. I'm not the same person I was ... I've changed. And I'm so afraid of getting hurt that I don't think I will ever be able to love again. Can you help me? Can anyone or anything help me? I just want to feel like 'me' again, not the empty shell I've become.

Please let me say how sorry I am for your loss. The death of someone we love deeply is recognized as one of the most traumatic, stressful and difficult experiences we ever face. The depth of your grief and the extent to which your partner's loss is still affecting you after almost three years, is evident from your letter.

You seem to have raised a number of issues in your letter, let's clearly identify them so we can explore them one-by-one. Firstly, you talk about your future and what it means to live a meaningful life. You also mention being 'mad with grief' and that you feel you've changed so much you don't feel like the same man you were before loss and grief changed your world forever. You say that you're afraid of being hurt again, and you ask whether anyone or anything can help you. Finally, you ask whether you will ever be able to love again?

I'm going to answer your questions in reverse. Many people do go on to meet someone and fall in love again after a bereavement, but everyone's period of grieving and recovery is slightly different, and there's no definitive timeframe. Only you will know when you feel emotionally ready to begin thinking about the possibility of meeting someone else.

Interestingly, I've noticed that often, we will meet someone before we really **feel** ready, and the process of getting to know them, and in time, perhaps learning to love them, is one of the things that helps to heal our hearts.

I understand why you think your experience has changed you so much that you don't feel you're the same person you used to be. You won't be; all of our experience changes us, whether that's love or loss. I wish that I could offer you an assurance that you won't ever be hurt again, but I can't. There are no guarantees with either love or relationships, although I will suggest that both are worth the risk when we feel that we've met the right person.

You ask whether anyone or anything can help you? Yes, of course. There are professional therapists who will support you if you ask them to. You will also find that your friends and family will support you, even if you've withdrawn yourself from them over the past few years. If you reach out to them I'm sure that they will respond with love, as our connections with others make our lives meaningful and your wellbeing will be important to them.

There are a number of things which make our lives meaningful. Very often our work is one of them and of course our relationships are another. So too is kindness; doing things which help others can be hugely rewarding. This is magnified when the things we do also connect us to some kind of a sense of purpose; i.e. acting in accordance with our values for a reason greater than ourselves.

Because of your loss, your life will never be the same again. You will have to learn to live your life differently and to rebuild it. Please use your love for your partner to give you strength and at some time in the future I'm sure you will eventually feel ready to live and to love again.

Epilogue

It's my greatest hope that this book will make a positive difference to you in some way. Whether that's new self-knowledge which contributes to your self-awareness, information which helps you develop your relationships with other people, or insights which will prompt you to change the ways you think and work. All are equally as valuable and will help you to embrace more Love in your life.

There's a lot of new information within these pages, and probably some scientific research which you won't have come across before. So you may find yourself reading certain parts of the book more than once. Also, if you experience any significant changes within your life, you might find it useful to complete your Love Life Audit again too. Remember that sometimes, not everything has to change for everything to change.

Many people seem to think that personal development is a one-off; that we can go on a workshop or read a few of the 'right' books and that's it. But if you're reading this book, you and I know something quite different. We know that personal development isn't a one-off event; it's an attitude, and more than that, it's a journey of self-awareness and often spiritual enlightenment, which lasts a lifetime.

There is no doubt that recognising, and bringing, more Love into your life, especially Healthy Self-Love, will make you feel better physically and emotionally. It will subtly alter how you feel about yourself and other people, and as a result, your world will change. More than that, the world will be a much better place for having you in it; as, day by day, you make a difference in your own way.

I would encourage you to practice mindfulness and Loving Kindness Meditation. In fact, I would encourage you to do all of those things which will engage your vagus nerve and prompt the release of oxytocin. It's profoundly healing; Love really is The Answer.

Notes and References

Chapter 2

The following resources all relate to our current understanding of the Vagus Nerve:

Trust Your Gut – There's Nothing Woo-Woo About the Vagus Nerve. Christopher Bergland, The Athlete's Way. Freely available on *www.psychologytoday.com*

Why the Vagus Nerve is so Important. Jordan Rosenfeld. On *www.mentalfloss.com*

How Does the Vagus Nerve Convey Gut Instincts to the Brain? Christopher Bergland, The Athlete's Way. Freely available on *www.psychologytoday.com*

Gut Vagal Afferents Differentially Modulate Innate Anxiety and Learned Fear. May 2014, Journal of Neuroscience.

Chapter 2 - References

1. B. Fredrickson et al., (2008). Open hearts build lives: positive increases in emotions, induced through loving-kindness meditation, build consequential resources. *Journal of Personality and Social Psychology*, 95, (5), pp.1,045-62.

2. J. W. Carson et al., (2005). Loving-kindness meditation for chronic low back pain. *Journal of Holistic Nursing*, 23, (3), pp.287-304.

3. T. G. Plante & C. E. Thorensen, (2007). *Spirit, Science and Health: How the Spiritual Mind Fuels Physical Wellness.* Praeger Publishers: Westport.

4. S. W. Lazare et al., (2005). Meditation experience is associated with increased cortical thickness. *Neuroreport*, 16, pp.893-7.

5. T. Singer & T. Lamm, (2009). The Social Neuroscience of Empathy. *Annals of the New York Academy of Sciences*, 1, (156), pp.81-96.

6. G. Hein & T. Singer, (2008). I feel how you feel but not always: the empathetic brain and its modulation. *Current Opinion in Neurobiology*, 18, pp.153-8.

7. C. Bergland, (2013). *The 'Love Hormone' Drives Human Urge for Social Connection*, on www.Psychologytoday.com

8. Dolen, G., et al., (2013). Social Reward Requires Coordinated Activity of Nucleus Accumbens Oxytocin and Serotonin. *Nature*, 12;501(7466):179-84. doi:10.1038/nature12518.

9. V. B, Mornhenn et al., (2007). Monetary sacrifice among strangers is mediated by endogenous oxytocin release after physical contact. *Evolution and Human Behaviour*, 29, pp.375-83.

10. J. A. Silvers & J. Haidt, (2008). Moral elevation can induce nursing. *Emotion*, 8, (2), pp.291-5.

11. T. Baumgartner et al., (2008). Oxytocin shapes the neural circuitry of trust and trust adaptation in humans. *Neuron*, 58, pp.639-50.

12. E. Callaway, (2009). Love hormone boosts strangers' sex appeal. *New Scientist*, 9th April. Freely available from *https://www.newscientist.com/article/dn16932-love-hormone-boosts-strangers-sex-appeal/*

13. B. Ohlsson & S. Janciauskiene, (2007). New insights into the understanding of gastrointestinal dysmotility. *Drug Targets Insights*, 2, pp.229-37.

14. B. Ohlsson et al., (2004). Oxytocin stimulates colonic motor activity in healthy women. *Neurogastroenterology and Motility*, 16, pp.233-40.

15. A. Szeto et al., (2008). Oxytocin attenuates NADP-dependent superoxide activity and IL-6 secretion in macrophages and vascular cells. *American Journal of Endocrinology and Metabolism*, 295, (E1), pp.495-501.

16. T. W. Smith et al., (2006). Marital conflict behaviour and coronary artery calcification. Paper presented at the American Society's 64th Annual Meeting in Denver, Colorado, USA.

17. M. G. Cattaneo et al., (2009). Oxytocin stimulates in vitro angiogenesis via a Pyk-2/Src-dependent mechanism. *Experimental Cell Research*, 315, (18, 3), pp.210-19.

18. A. Luks, (1991). *The Healing Power of Doing Good*. See *www.IUniverse.com*

19. P. A. Thoits & L. N. Hewitt, (2001). Volunteer work and well-being, *Journal of Health and Social Behaviour*, 42, (2), pp.115-31.

20. M. A. Musick & J. Wilson, (2003). Volunteering and depression: the role of psychological and social resources in different age groups. *Social Science and Medicine*, 56, (2), pp.259-69.

21. E. A. Greenfield & N. F. Marks, (2004). Formal volunteering as a protective factor for older adults' psychological well-being. Journal of Gerontololgy Series B, *Psychological Sciences and Social Sciences*, 59, (5), pp.S258-64.

22. D. Oman, C. E. Thoresen & K. McMahon, (1999). Volunteerism and mortality among the community dwelling elderly. *Journal of Health Psychology*, 4. (3), pp.301-16.

23. H. S. Harris & C. E. Thoresen, (2005). Volunteering is associated with delayed mortality in older people: analysis of the longitudinal study of aging. *Journal of Health Psychology*, 10, (6), pp.739-62.

24. Candace Pert, (1997), Molecules of Emotion. Scribner.

25. C. Pert et al., (1980). Neuropeptides and their receptors: a psychosomatic network. *Journal of Immunology*, 135, (2), pp.820-26.

26. For more information, see 'Triune Brain Theory'.

27. B. Fredrickson, & B. Kok, (2013). How Positive Emotions Build Physical Health: Perceived Social Connections Account for Upward Spiral Between Positive Emotions and Vagal Tone. *Psychological Science*, 24, (7), pp.1123-32.

28. F. A. Coopman et al., (2016). Vagus Nerve Stimulation Inhibits Cykotine Production and Attenuates Disease Severity in Rheumatoid Arthritis. *Proceedings of the National Academy of Sciences*, (PSAS), 113, (29), pp.8284-9. Available at pnas.org

29. C. Bergland, (2016), Vagus Nerve Stimulation Dramatically Reduces Inflammation. *PsychologyToday.com*

30. J. M. Huston et al., (2007). Transcutaneous vagus nerve stimulation reduces serum high mobility group box 1 levels and improves survival in murine sepsis. *Critical Care Medicine*, 35, (12), 2, pp.762-8.

31. K. McGowan, (2007). Can we cure aging? http://discovermagazine.com/2007/dec/can-we-cure-aging and see A. Aviv, (2004). Telomeres and human aging: facts and fibs. *Science of Aging Knowledge Environment*, 51, p.43.

32. V. Chandra et al., (1983). The impact on marital status on survival after an acute myocardial infarction: a population study. *Journal of Epistemology*, 117, pp.320-25.

33. M. M. Weissman, (1987). Advances in psychiatric epidemiology: rates and risks for major depression. *American Journal of Public Health*, 77, pp.445-51.

34. K. D. O'Leary et al., (1994). A closer look at the link between marital discord and depressive symptomatology. *Journal of Social and Clinical Psychology*, 13, pp.33-41.

35. C. K. Ewart et al., (1991). High blood pressure and marital discord: not being nasty matters more than being nice. *Health Psychology*, 10, pp.153-63.

36. J. K. Kiecolt-Glaser et al., (1993). Negative behaviour during marital conflict is associated with immunological down-regulation. *Psychosomatic Medicine*, 55, pp.395-409.

37. W. Malarkey et al., (1994). Hostile behaviour during marital conflict alters pituitary and adrenal hormones. *Psychosomatic Medicine*, 56, pp.41-51.

38. J. K. Kiecolt-Glaser et al., (1997). Marital conflict in older adults: endocrinological and immunological correlates. *Psychosomatic Medicine*, 59, pp.339-49.

39. J. K. Kiecolt-Glaser et al., (2005). Hostile marital relations, pro-inflammatory cycotine production and wound healing. *Archives of General Psychiatry*, 62, (12), pp.1377-84.

40. E. Sjogren et al., (2006). Interleukin-6 levels in relation to psychosocial factors: studies on serum, saliva and in-vitro production by blood mononuclear cells. *Brain Behaviour and Immunity*, 20, pp.270-78.

41. C. E. Detillon et al., (2004).   Social facilitation of wound healing. *Psychoneuroendocrinology*, 29, (8), pp.1004-11.

42. A. Vitalo et al., (2009). Nest making and oxytocin comparability promote wound healing in isolated reared rats. *http://dx.doi.org/10.1371/journal.pone.0005523*

43. B. Ditzen et al., (2008). Positive couple interactions and daily cortisol: on the stress-protecting role of intimacy. *Psychosomatic Medicine*, 70, pp.883-9.

44. T. Seeman et al., (1994). Social ties and support and neuroendocrine function: the MacArthur studies of successful aging. *Annals of Behavioral Medicine*, 16, pp.95-106.

45. K. Uvnas-Moberg, (1998). Oxytocin may mediate the benefits of positive social interactions and emotions. *Psychoneuroendocrinology*, 23, pp.819-35.

46. E Callaway, *New Scientist*, 14 January 2009, Pet dogs rival humans for emotional satisfaction. Freely available from *https://www.newscientist.com/arRcle/dn16412-pet-dogs-rival-humans-for-emotional-satisfaction/*

47. Mimi Guarneri, (2006). *The Heart Speaks*, Simon & Schuster.

48. E. J. Langer & J. Rodin, (1976). The effects of choice and enhanced social responsibility for the aged: a field experiment in an institutional setting. *Journal of Personality and Social Psychology*, 34, (2), pp.191-8.

49. M. Tops et al. (2007). Individual differences in emotional expressivity predict oxytocin responses to cortisol administration: relevance to breast cancer? *Biological Psychology*, 75, (2), pp.119-23.

50. R. White-Traut et al., (2009). Detection of salivary oxytocin levels in lactating women. *Developmental Psychobiology*, 51, (4), pp.367-73.

51. Holt-Lunstad et al., (2008). Influence of a 'warm touch' support enhancement intervention among married couples on ambulatory blood pressure, oxytocin, alpha amylase and cortisol. *Psychosomatic Medicine*, 70, pp.976-85.

52. K. C. Light et al., (2005). More frequent partner hugs and higher oxytocin levels are linked to lower blood pressure and heart rate in premenopausal women. *Biological Psychology*, 69, pp.5-21.

Chapter 3

1. Keeping hand submerged in iced water experiments for family love. Reference unavailable at this time.

1. *It Pays to Play*, (April 2016), from Bright HR, freely available to download from *www.brighthr.com*

2. Steffens N., et al.,(2016). A Meta-Analytic Review of Social Identification and Health in Organisational Contexts. *Personality and Social Psychology Review*, 1-33, cited by Jake Matthews on HR Grapevine, 14 October 2916, *'Why you should encourage banter in the workplace'*, see *www.hrgrapevine.com*

3. Kugler, L. & Kuhbandner, C., (2015). That's not funny! – But it should be: effects of humorous emotion regulation on emotional experience and memory. Frontiers in Psychology, 6, PMID 26379608. Cited in, 'The comforting power of comedy is due to more than just distraction', by David Robson on the BPS Digest, 2015, freely available on *www.digest.bps.org.uk*

4. *No, being kind to yourself does not make you weak or immodest.* Christian Jarrett, 27th May, 2016, freely available on *www.digest.bps.org.uk*

5. Lee Randall, *For the Love of Stuff*. Available via my twitter feed, @fionabedjones

6. Ulrich, R. S., (1984). View through a window may influence recovery from surgery. *Science*, vol. 224, p.420 (2), pp.1-3.

Chapter 5
1. Lee Randall, *For the Love of Stuff*. Available via my twitter feed, *@fionabedjones*

Chapter 7
1. S. Lyubomirsky, C. Tkach & K. M. Sheldon, (2004). *Pursuing sustained happiness through random acts of kindness*, University of California, Riverside, Department of Psychology. Cited by David R. Hamilton, (2010), *Why Kindness is Good For You*, p.237, UK: HayHouse.

2. Gordon, G., (2014). Well Played. The origins and future of playfulness. *American Journal of Play*, 6, (2), pp.234-266. Freely available from *http://files.eric.ed.gov/fulltext/EJ1023802.pdf*

3. T. Seeman et al., (1994). Social ties and support and neuroendocrine function: the MacArthur studies of successful aging. Annals of Behavioral Medicine, 16, pp.95-106.

4. T. W. Smith et al., (2006). Marital conflict behaviour and coronary artery calcification. Paper presented at the American Society's 64th Annual Meeting in Denver, Colorado, USA.

5. V. Chandra et al., (1983). The impact on marital status on survival after an acute myocardial Infarction: a population study. *Journal of Epistemology*, 117, pp.320-25.

6. M. M. Weissman, (1987). Advances in psychiatric epidemiology: rates and risks for major depression. *American Journal of Public Health*, 77, pp.445-51.

7. K. D. O'Leary et al., (1994). A closer look at the link between marital discord and depressive symptomatology. *Journal of Social and Clinical Psychology*, 13, pp.33-41.

8. C. K. Ewart et al., (1991). High blood pressure and marital discord: not being nasty matters more than being nice. *Health Psychology*, 10, pp.153-63.

9. J. K. Kiecolt-Glaser et al., (1993). Negative behaviour during marital conflict is associated with immunological down-regulation. *Psychosomatic Medicine*, 55, pp.395-409.

10. W. Malarkey et al., (1994). Hostile behaviour during marital conflict alters pituitary and adrenal hormones. *Psychosomatic Medicine*, 56, pp.41-51.

11. J. K. Kiecolt-Glaser et al., (1997). Marital conflict in older adults: endocrinological and immunological correlates. *Psychosomatic Medicine*, 59, pp.339-49.

12. J. K. Kiecolt-Glaser et al., (2005). Hostile marital relations, pro-inflammatory cycotine production and wound healing. *Archives of General Psychiatry*, 62, (12), pp.1377-84.

Chapter 8

1. Sisodia, R. et al., (2007). *Firms of Endearment: How World-Class Companies Profit from Passion and Purpose*. Wharton School Publishing.

2. Beddoes-Jones, F., (2016). *Divided by Gender, United by Chocolate: Differences in the Boardroom.* Blue Ocean Publishing. Also see *www.unitedbychocolate.com*

The Leadership Temperament Types™ questionnaire and report are available directly from *www.unitedbychocolate.com* as are details of Training and Licensing Workshops for its use within organisations.

3. Beddoes-Jones, F., (2009). *Thinking Styles – Relationship Strategies That Work!* BJA Associates Ltd. Also see *www.cognitivefitness.co.uk*

The Thinking Styles™ questionnaire and report are available from The Cognitive Fitness Consultancy, as is information on training and licensing for its use within organisations.

About the Author

Dr Fiona Beddoes-Jones is a leadership development professional and Executive Coach who specialises in helping individuals and teams achieve extraordinary things. She is a Chartered Psychologist and regularly speaks at international conferences in the areas of:

- Leadership Temperament Types
- Authentic Leadership and Leadership Development
- Teamwork and Extraordinary Performance
- Cognitive Fitness and Cognitive Team Roles
- Leading and Managing Volunteers
- Developing Effective Relationships
- The Corporate Love Model

Fiona is the author of the psychometric instruments Thinking Styles™, Cognitive Team Roles™ and the UK's only Authentic Leadership 360, developed with the UK's Royal Air Force.

As well as her corporate work, Fiona also runs personal development workshops on Love Is The Answer for people who want to explore the Love they currently have in their lives and to recreate their future in a safe and supportive environment.

In her spare time, Fiona is a volunteer Environmental Ranger at Rutland Water. She is also the Race Psychologist for the UK's annual ultra-endurance marathon, The Spine Race as well as being Expedition Psychologist for the Ice Warrior Project.

Other books by Dr Fiona Beddoes-Jones:
- Divided by Gender, United by Chocolate: Differences in the Boardroom
- Thinking Styles – Relationship Strategies That Work!
- Jane Eyre's Rival: The Real Mrs Rochester

A full list of articles, publications and conference presentations by Fiona is available from *www.cognitivefitness.co.uk*